I0418444

The Crane and the Grandmaster

By

Darryl Vidal

Copyright © 2025 Darryl Vidal.

All rights reserved. No part of this book may be reproduced, distributed, or transmitted in any form without written permission from the author.

Table of Contents

Foreword

There are moments in our lives when film transcends entertainment and becomes transformative and impactful. That moment came in 1984 when I sat down in a Bronx movie theatre with my mother and toddler sister to watch a film that would become the compass of my youth—The Karate Kid.

The story of a young man learning to navigate a complex world through lessons of discipline, respect, and inner strength, spoke directly to my circumstances and needs. I wasn't just following Daniel LaRusso's journey—I was using it as a roadmap to navigate my own course.

Growing up in a single-parent household without a father figure and struggling with abandonment issues created a monumental void. The Karate Kid impacted me emotionally. I wasn't just watching a movie about martial arts; I was searching for guidance and a mentor. The film gave me hope that I could one day meet a Mr. Miyagi figure who would provide those priceless lessons passed down from generation to generation.

The scene that made Mr. Miyagi feel credible as a lifelong student and teacher who tied the ancient traditions of martial arts with his mentoring of Daniel was when he was standing gracefully on that California beach stump at sunset, executing what we would all come to know as the iconic Crane Kick.

At that moment, the philosophy became physical. The fiction became authentic. What I didn't know then—what none of us casual viewers knew back in 1984—was the figure that stood on that stump wasn't the older man with grey and thinning hair; it was a young man who was on the same path of the fictional Miyagi, dedicating his life to his craft and sharing his knowledge with those that sought it out. The soul of that authenticity had a name: Darryl Vidal.

A few years later, when technology finally delivered a VCR, I would spend hours rewinding and replaying the tournament scenes featuring "Vidal," studying his extraordinary kicks and displays of martial arts mastery with a mixture of awe and determination. His presence in those scenes conveyed something that no script could manufacture: the genuine spirit of karate, honed through years of disciplined practice.

With the innocent skepticism of youth, I remember wondering how Johnny Lawrence could have advanced past such a formidable opponent; how was "Vidal" not the undisputed All-Valley Karate Champion? The argument,

Copyright © 2025 Darryl Vidal

and our poor attempts to reenact "Vidal's" moves, would go on for many years between me and my childhood friends.

Life has a remarkable way of completing circles we never knew we were drawing. In 2020, nearly four decades after that transformative theater experience, I found myself collaborating with Darryl on a project aimed at amplifying the stories of underrepresented voices—including Asian American Pacific Islanders.

Having become an unofficial historian of The Karate Kid, I was intimately familiar with Darryl's film and pop culture contributions. The Crane Kick has become a part of American culture; there's a good chance somebody will mimic the infamous kick whenever there is playful banter related to fighting. While our project ultimately didn't materialize, a friendship formed through our shared belief in the power of authentic storytelling.

In the years since, I've continued to encourage Darryl to share his unique journey. The man who delivered one of cinema's most recognizable moments has lived a life rich with wisdom that extends far beyond that beach scene or tournament floor. He has dedicated over 50 years of his life to practicing martial arts and sharing his knowledge and experience with thousands of students; his story encompasses not just the technical mastery of martial arts but the philosophical depth that gives those moves meaning.

The book you hold in your hands is not a memoir or some type of martial arts manual. It is the culmination of a lifetime dedicated to an art form that teaches us as much about understanding life's challenges as it does about the journey of a young man who had an unwavering commitment to martial arts and helped build the foundation for a timeless story that continues to live on.

It is the wisdom of a student who understood that before "Daniel-San" could learn to punch or kick, he needed to learn to wax cars, paint fences and a house, and sand a deck—the fundamental truth is that building character is the first step to building skill.

For those who, like me, found direction and more profound meaning through The Karate Kid, this book offers a deeper understanding of the authenticity that made the film resonate across generations. For those new to Darryl's story, it presents an opportunity to learn about someone who has lived the principles that most of us have only encountered through fiction and has shared them with countless students over a half-century.

As you turn these pages, know that you're receiving guidance from the same spirit that once stood on that beach stump, demonstrating what balance and a strong work ethic truly means—both in martial arts and in life.

Robert Vazquez
Unofficial Karate Kid Historian and Friend to Darryl Vidal

Copyright © 2025 Darryl Vidal

Introducing, Me!

Hello, I'm Darryl. That's how I usually introduce myself. I like to follow tradition. A strong handshake and eye-to-eye contact—which is even more important for short people. I like to squeeze their hand just enough to leave a mild impression. Of course, if it's someone dating my daughter I squeeze much harder, and look right through them.

Always stand up and speak clearly. Show deference to your new acquaintance. You never know, you may be meeting a prince or a CEO or an important celebrity—and even if they're not, there's nothing wrong with treating people nicely, no matter what.

Try not to take over the conversation, but be an active participant. Listen closely and show interest, as much as possible.

One of my issues when meeting new people is mostly about context. I do a lot of different things, you might say I wear a lot of hats, so if I meet someone on the street, I usually stop with , "My name is Darryl," and wait for some sort of context to focus the conversation. I get bored with some conversations very quickly, and sometimes I can't hide it, to negative effect. It's one of the things I continue to work on socially.

It might just end there, where we talk about the weather or traffic or other innocuous subject matter. I typically won't dive right into something unless I have a motive or objective. I'm usually hesitant to take the discussion in any particular direction so I don't hijack the conversation.

It's actually not that I think that I'm so interesting, but at any given time or place, I don't like to be the person to take over a conversation. The circumstances of the introduction will often dictate, if it's my meeting, then I will definitely take control of the conversation. In a business situation I'm very cognizant of my role and objective in a meeting and I will adhere to it as much as possible.

Since I'm typically the client in most of my current business, I'm always aware of the cards that I hold. Being the client means that "I'm always right" and I'm the one seeking satisfaction. It's just as common however that I am managing a project for another department, in which case they are the client. That doesn't mean that I don't direct the discussion, only that I am the one seeking their satisfaction.

Unfortunately, I'm not a big sports fan. I like to watch football (American), and even some baseball (mostly highlights). So I'm pretty lame when people are talking about their fantasy football team. I like to watch Formula 1 racing and I love to watch and play golf, so there's that.

I can be pretty bold at times, or self-indulgent. Maybe even a little narcissistic. Not so much conceited these days; I was very conceited for most of my teenage years, before I learned to temper it and keep my mouth shut. I started to realize how overbearing it is to listen to someone talk about themself all the time and I could feel myself competing for attention. So I realized, this has to stop. Let people toot their horns. They will quickly fall out of the attention loop without my help.

I guess I'm a little quiet, or shy by nature. I would just rather go along with a conversation that someone else is directing. I'll let them inflate their ego so I don't. It's sort of a balancing act of awareness and self-promotion.

This actually took years of growing up, and self-examination to understand that people like to talk about things they are interested in. They get quickly bored or impatient with someone who has a conversational agenda.

But context can present itself quickly or by circumstance. If we meet at a martial arts tournament for instance, then it can be assumed we're going to be talking about karate or martial arts in some vein. In which case I will jump in to test the waters (conversationally).

Once again, to a more granular degree, this subject can also be delicate or politically charged (I'm referring to the politics of martial arts systems and lineage, which has tested loyalties and caused many feuds over the years).

But rarely would I start where most people who know me think I would start a conversation. I never bring up karate or my involvement in a movie, or my ranking unless it becomes a point of discussion. And if we get to martial arts, I'll ease into it. If they're asking about karate classes, I'll tell them what they need to know to stay interested. People don't want to take karate from me just because I was in a movie. They must see that I have a solid, fundamentals-based approach. I'll almost never bring up my rank unless specifically asked.

Why? You might ask? Because there's nothing more vain than saying, "I'm a 10th degree black belt." Or, "I'm a Grandmaster in Kenpo Karate." It's always better to do a leveling and have a discussion appropriate to the

Copyright © 2025 Darryl Vidal

participants. If it's a parent bragging about their 10 year old Black Belt, I always say, "Wow, that's an amazing accomplishment."

So if we were to meet in passing, on the street or at the market, you would never know about the Crane or the Grandmaster. It's just as well. It's more enthusiasm I'll have left for someone who's truly interested in these things. Which these days is a lot of people. People want to know about my style of karate, my rank, how I got started, etc., etc. So I do my best to be enthusiastic for these interviewers and podcasters. Nothing worse than listening to an interview where it's clear the interviewee is bored or disinterested.

Once these subjects are broached, I'll address the curiosity, but quickly take the discussion down a path to ensure we can all share interest.

There are some things I love to talk about in depth, like authors and books in the techno-thriller realm, outdoors, fishing, or any of a number of side-interests and hobbies I have. Here I can spend hours talking about the finest nuances and details.

I can discuss my golf index (even how legitimate it is), how to dual-haul a fly-fishing cast, or even how to accelerate out of a high-speed turn in a racing simulator. But similarly, I wouldn't walk down any of these paths without some impetus.

So, where to start a book about myself? As you might guess, it's not easy. How can you write a book about yourself without being boastful and narcissistic? It's true, most of my friends and acquaintances encourage me to write a book about my experiences, but it wasn't until my oldest son admonished me. "You have to have this ready for when you come out in Cobra Kai! You're going to blow up! People will want to know about you and your story." Thanks for the encouragement Justin!

I wrestled with my own identity for years contemplating this endeavor. It just seems so self-involved and self-indulgent. One knows how annoying it can be when people talk about themselves continuously. So this is the balance I seek. The image I portray. The act I put forward. You can act with humility, but it has to be part of your true nature for others to recognize it. That's why I always take it as the highest compliment to be described as a humble, modest person.

So, let's start at the beginning. I have to qualify this writing by stating that although I'm starting at the

Copyright © 2025 Darryl Vidal

beginning of my existence, it would be unnatural to strictly adhere to chronology. So this book may meander, but it's in my nature to follow the flow, just as in Filipino Martial Arts (FMA), we will go where the story takes us.

San Diego was my birthplace, but in my life, it is more than just a city; it is a symbol of the opportunities and challenges that came with being the only American-born member of my family. My older brothers were born in the Philippines, and our family's story was one of transition—from the rich cultural traditions of our homeland to the new, uncharted waters of American life. This distinction of being the only one born in the U.S. set me apart in a unique way, both within my family and in the broader context of our lives as an American among immigrant parents.

I was born on May 20, 1963, in San Diego, California, the youngest of three boys in a family that had only recently made its way to American shores. My parents, Roman and Belen Vidal, were Filipino immigrants who had embarked on a journey that would take them halfway around the world, eventually bringing them to the United States. My father's decision to join the US Navy as a kitchen steward was the catalyst for our family's relocation, and it was this choice that shaped much of my early life.

My father, Roman, had joined the US Navy not long before he and my mother were married. It was a decision that would bring a measure of stability to our family, but it also meant a life defined by movement. After arriving in San Diego, where I was born, we didn't stay in one place for long. My father's naval career took us from San Diego to Bremerton, Washington, then to Newport, Rhode Island, then back to San Diego.

Each move was a new chapter in our family's story, with its own set of challenges and adventures. In Rhode Island, I remember the lush green hills and the cool, warm damp air that was so different from the sun-soaked streets of San Diego.

Newport, Rhode Island, was a place where my brothers and I spent hours playing outside, exploring the natural beauty that surrounded our naval housing tract, near a railway. It was a time of discovery, both of the world around us and of our own identities as Filipino-Americans.

Some of my most vivid memories are of catching grasshoppers in the field and throwing stones near the railroad track. The concept of four seasons never made sense until these elementary school years.

We learned about snow and sledding, and staying warm at night. We saw the seasons change, trees dump their leaves and the colors and mud of Spring.

Newport, brought another change in scenery and culture. The East Coast was a world away from the West Coast, with its own pace of life and its own traditions. For my parents, it was another step in their journey to build a life in this new country. For me, it was a chance to experience the diversity of America firsthand from behind the most innocent eyes, to see how different places could be, yet still be part of the same country. Curiously, the event that stayed with me to this day was watching the moon landing in my kindergarten classroom. An appropriate memory based on historical significance.

After years of moving from place to place, we eventually returned to San Diego, where my father would complete his Navy career. San Diego became our home base, the place where our family finally put down roots. It was a return to the city that had first welcomed them to America. For me, it was a place of continuity, where I

Copyright © 2025 Darryl Vidal

could start to build my own identity. But that wouldn't last long either.

Growing up as the youngest of three boys in a new suburban tract neighborhood was both a blessing and a challenge. I was a small, thin child, yet my wiry frame belied the athleticism that surged within me. My days were filled with the joyous chaos of street baseball and football, games that brought together all the kids in our neighborhood. The sounds of laughter, the thud of a ball hitting a glove, and the cheers of a well-played game were the soundtrack of my youth. We rode our bikes to the ditches and watched the new tract homes spring up all around us.

But life wasn't without its challenges. I battled asthma, a condition that often left me feeling frustrated and limited. The wheeze in my chest would remind me that my body wasn't invincible. Yet, even in those moments of discomfort, I refused to let my ailments define me. I was determined to push through, to prove to myself and to others that I was capable of great things despite the obstacles in my way. The drive to overcome this challenge became a defining part of my character, shaping my resilience and fortitude.

My parents and brothers had all been born in the Philippines, bringing with them the traditions and cultural heritage of their homeland. Our home was filled with the sounds, smells, and customs of the Philippines with an interesting mix of Americana, from the vibrant music that played during family gatherings to the delicious aroma of traditional dishes simmering on the stove, intermixed with the music of Elvis, and Chubby Checker, pizza and hamburgers mixed in with Tinikling, pancit and lumpia. I was deeply connected to this heritage, yet I was also acutely aware of my role as a bridge between two worlds.

Being born in America gave me a unique perspective, one that was different from my brothers. I straddled the line between the old world and the new, between the traditions of our Filipino heritage and the opportunities of American life.

I carried with me the values and lessons passed down from my parents, the respect for elders, the importance of family, and the deep sense of the need to study and excel in school that was central to our Filipino identity. This duality shaped my worldview, making me both a product of my environment and a future custodian of my heritage; something I was yet to define. Yet ironically, none of us

Copyright © 2025 Darryl Vidal

learned the native language of the country, Tagalog. In my parents' effort to Americanize themselves, they spoke English in the house.

The interesting thing about Asian families and their work ethic through education is somewhat unguided. It was assumed that you will do well in classes so you can go to college. The whole thing about what you will do once there was never significantly discussed or promoted. But that's okay, as long as we were okay following the prescribed path to success; the American Dream.

My father's journey through the Navy ranks was a testament to his determination and adaptability. Starting as a kitchen steward in a predominantly Filipino environment, since he had college credits in Engineering he broke through the ranks to train in the Machinery Repairman rating. The Machinery Repairman (MR) rating in the U.S. Navy is a technical rating within the engineering field. Sailors in this rating are skilled machinists responsible for repairing, maintaining, and fabricating metal parts and machinery. They are trained in operating machine tools such as lathes, milling machines, grinders, and drill presses to create or repair parts needed for various naval systems.

He became a respected member of the Machinery Repair rating successfully ascending to Master Chief (E-9). This accomplishment not only defined his career but also significantly impacted his social circle.

As my father ascended the ranks, he found himself immersed in a new world of American sailors and their families. The parties we attended were a fascinating blend of cultures, where Filipino traditions met American customs. The food, music, and conversations reflected the diverse backgrounds of the attendees. It was a place where people from different walks of life could come together and celebrate their shared experiences. The phenomenon of White men with Asian wives was so commonplace, it seemed to be a thing.

The exposure to this new social circle had a profound influence on me as a child. I grew up surrounded by people of various ethnicities and backgrounds, which helped to shape my understanding of society. I learned to appreciate the beauty of diversity and to embrace the richness of different cultures.

What mattered most about my father's success was that it was all simple and straightforward. Do well, and represent yourself well. He was also a great

Copyright © 2025 Darryl Vidal

do-it-yourselfer, which ultimately made him a successful landlord. Although I can't say I'm as handy as he was, I can say that I have a keen understanding of what I can do within my semi-skilled means and what I should leave to a professional.

My father was a driven man. He never dilly dallied. One of the reasons we weren't a sports family was likely because he didn't think American sports were a valuable pastime—even a waste of time. Of course, this is something he would only say within the walls of our home. He was much too shrewd to say something like that in public.

He was a deal maker. In whatever was his current hobby or distraction, he would learn the ins and outs and look to find value in the transaction. Some of the best lessons in deal making I learned watching him at garage sales and swap meets. In my mom's words he was more or less a "junk collector" buying random items and reselling them at the swap meet.

The family spent a few Saturdays at the local swap meet and I can recall him coming home with wads of cash—maybe $2-$3,000, which is a lot of cash to have in your pocket in the 80's. Then the next weekend we'd be out hitting all the garage sales first thing the next morning, parlaying the cash into new treasures to store in the junk pile until the next swap meet adventure.

My favorite story of how driven he could be was early one Saturday morning while garage saleing. There was a large mirror he wanted to buy—4 feet by 8 feet. He was in his Honda Prelude so he called me from home to help him load the mirror into my truck. In those days he had to ask the homeowner if he could use the phone and I was at home sleeping.

I went to the garage sale location and we picked up the mirror, each of us holding our side to load it carefully into the truck. As we turned the mirror, it hit the truck sidewall and cracked down the middle.

Large triangular shard of broken mirror lanced down his chest cutting a ragged hole in his white t-shirt. One thing my dad always did was dress like he was poor when garage saleing. He said, if you show off like you're rich, no one will give you a deal. Better to look poor when making deals. Not true for all transaction types but you can definitely understand the reasoning—what I call shrewd.

Anyway, the mirror was broken into a thousand pieces and his chest was bleeding from what looked like a surface wound, even though it started bleeding profusely. We tended to his wound but he felt it wasn't too deep, he could drive himself to the emergency room, since we had both vehicles. I told him I would meet him there.

I got to the hospital before him and waited (no cell phones). Half an hour later, he shows up at the ER covered in blood.

"Where were you!" I admonished. I was worried I'd have to go look for him only to find him crashed out on the road bleeding to death. He said, "I stopped at two more garage sales! Boy did they look at me funny!"

I was always the most like my dad. He had dark skin unlike my mother and my brothers. They had the lighter skin that was more desirable. Not only did we share that trait, face and body-type, I was truly his mini-me. Even as I'm in my 60s, I look exactly like him. He had a great sense of humor, but when got into his late 30's, it was as if he was training me to be his comedic sidekick.

Since I was pretty good and doing card tricks and memorizing things, he would have me "perform" these tricks and tell jokes to all his Navy buddies. He actually would buy these joke books, which could never be

Copyright © 2025 Darryl Vidal

published today, and I would memorize the jokes, and repeat them to his friends like a vaudeville act.

I can't even imagine today, some little Asian kid telling these terrible Polish and Jewish jokes in front of a bunch of Navy Chiefs.

It really helped me develop a sense for puns and comedic timing—and I can still rattle off many of those off-color jokes he had me telling, but only in the most guarded company.

Being Filipino by heritage and American by birth, I found myself navigating a complex balancing act. When my family moved from San Diego to Chino, a predominantly white and Hispanic community, I experienced a stark contrast in diversity from Mira Mesa—where Navy Filipino families were common. There were only one or two other Filipino students in the school, making me feel like an outsider.

It was also amusing that because I was Asian it was assumed that I knew martial arts. Most of my classmates didn't even know what Filipino was. I was usually asked if I was Chinese or Japanese.

The irony wasn't lost on me. Here I was, an Asian kid in a predominantly white school, expected to be a martial arts master. It was as if my ethnicity was a prerequisite for knowing how to break boards and deliver flying kicks. Of course, I knew only the limited stick-fighting and karate that Vince had taught me. My Filipino heritage, while rich in culture, was largely unknown to my classmates.

Later that year, I found myself on the other side of this cultural misunderstanding. A new Asian student arrived, and I, in my infinite wisdom, proceeded to quiz him about his nationality. "Chinese, Japanese, Vietnamese, Filipino, Thai?" I rattled off, my mind ticking off the possibilities. To my embarrassment, he revealed he was Korean. It was a classic case of assuming everyone else's ethnicity is as exotic and obscure as your own.

Then, when we had wrestling together we compared notes on if either knew martial arts.

We shared a laugh over our stereotypical experience, both of us victims of the same tired stereotypes. It was a moment of unexpected camaraderie, a reminder that despite our differences, we were both just trying to navigate the complexities of high school life.

Copyright © 2025 Darryl Vidal

Musically

In our household, talent was never in short supply. My older brothers, Irwin and Vinci (whom I will refer to as Vince often), were both gifted musicians who would carve out their niches in the arts. Irwin started with the piano, his fingers playing Beethoven and Mozart, while Vince mastered the accordion, producing rich, polka melodies. But their musical journeys didn't stop there. Irwin, ever the self-learner, went on to teach himself guitar, while Vinci, with his natural ear for sound, could pick up any brass instrument—whether it was the French horn or the saxophone—and play it with ease.

When my father bought a drum set, neither of them had any formal training, yet both could sit down and play as if they'd been practicing for years. It was as though music lived in their veins, a second language they both spoke fluently.

Once playing the drums, Vinci moved from the horn section to the drum line of the marching band. Ours was the house where the kids would come over and we'd have the radio cranked up loud and one of my brothers would be playing the drums along with whatever was playing. If it

Copyright © 2025 Darryl Vidal

were another day, Irwin would also have his electric guitar and amp and the house would be jamming for hours on end.

For me, however, the science of music didn't seem to manifest in the same way. I understood and could feel the music, but I wasn't getting the formal training.

While I envied their abilities, watching them create music from instruments and notes on a page I couldn't replicate what came so naturally to them.

I sat at the piano with no guidance struggling to count the lines of the treble clef and banged on the drums without the steady tempo and bass kick that mimicked the music played over the radio. I knew the mechanics, but did not commit to any specific instrument. Their passion was palpable, their connection to music undeniable. Music was their language, their expression. Not so, for little brother.

It was with one of their first attempts to create a rock and roll band that someone had left a bass and bass amp at our house for a few months. It was then I learned the most rudimentary of bass playing and started realizing I wasn't completely unmusical; just mostly unmusical.

It wasn't until my later teenage years that I discovered I had some musical potential of my own. Irwin, patient and encouraging, took the time to teach me the most basic guitar barre chords. As I practiced, something clicked, and I realized I did have a latent talent after all—rhythm. I found that I could strum intricate and complex beat patterns with ease, and I had a decent sense of timing.

Learning to play the bass by focusing on fretboard patterns rather than reading notes transformed music from a complex language of symbols into something tactile and accessible. I learned early on that the bass fretboard is essentially laid out in the pentatonic scale, a pattern that made navigating notes feel more like a physical roadmap. This allowed me to tap into my strength in pattern recognition rather than traditional music theory, following familiar shapes and relationships on the neck. Even though I didn't read music or have perfect pitch (not even decent pitch), I was able to let rhythm and intuition guide my fingers to the right places, building a feel for the groove and timing without needing to intellectualize every note.

This approach not only allowed me to play effectively at a rudimentary level, but also to write my own (simplistic) songs. Recognizing the simplicity and adaptability of the pentatonic scale, I could experiment with phrasing and timing to create unique rhythms and lines. By focusing on these patterns, I could hear the bass' potential as both a rhythmic and melodic instrument, shaping songs that reflected my style and approach.

It wasn't the same natural fluency my brothers had, but it was a discovery that gave me enough confidence to know that if I practice I will improve. Slowly, I began to appreciate that, while my path with music was different from my brothers, it was still uniquely mine.

High School

My freshman year of high school was a whirlwind of new experiences and academic challenges. Despite my natural abilities, I struggled with time management and procrastination. As a result, I earned a C in my first-quarter algebra classes, which significantly hampered my chances of achieving a perfect 4.0 GPA.

I wasn't going to let that happen again. School was typically so easy, all I needed to do was pay attention and I could surely get at least a B in every class.

Despite my uncertainty, I always had a strong sense that I was destined for something significant. I couldn't explain it, but there was a quiet confidence within me, a belief that I was meant to achieve good things in some way. Perhaps it was a coping mechanism, a way to navigate the feelings of inadequacy that sometimes crept in when I compared myself to my brothers. Or maybe it was a genuine intuition, a spark of insight that told me I had something unique to offer the world.

Into my late teens, this sense of purpose became more pronounced. I started to see my challenges not as burdens, but as opportunities to prove my strength and determination. Every time I pushed through a challenge, it felt like a small victory, a step closer to realizing my potential. These experiences taught me that life's difficulties could be overcome, that they were not insurmountable obstacles but rather tests of character. I began to see myself as someone who could rise above, who could achieve something meaningful despite the odds.

Imposter syndrome is a tricky mental balancing act, and for me, it felt like a tug-of-war between confidence and self-doubt. Even as I found talents and skills that set me apart, I couldn't fully enjoy them without that persistent sense of inadequacy countering the sense of pride. I didn't know it as "imposter syndrome" back then; I just thought of it as a yin-yang effect. Whenever I felt gifted or accomplished, those feelings seemed to immediately invite their opposite—a wave of self-doubt that would convince

Copyright © 2025 Darryl Vidal

me I might just be fooling everyone. Or more likely, just myself.

I was stuck in this cycle where any notion of being "special" was met with an equally powerful thought that I wasn't good enough and would never be.

I learned to live with this internal push-and-pull, letting each side temper the other. Sometimes, this humility was useful, keeping me grounded and constantly pushing me to work harder. But there were also times when this undercurrent of inadequacy felt more like a handicap, keeping me from fully embracing my abilities or accomplishments. I would find myself comparing my achievements to those of others, always convinced that someone else was more skilled, more deserving, or better prepared than I was. It was hard to know if I was genuinely talented or if I had just stumbled into success by luck or timing.

Looking back, I can see how imposter syndrome shaped my experiences and my approach to challenges. It meant I rarely took anything for granted and always felt I had to earn my place, whether in martial arts, music, or my career. Yet, it also sometimes held me back, creating a barrier to truly acknowledging what I was capable of. It was always there as an excuse to not commit or not execute. It fed procrastination.

Recognizing this balance as imposter syndrome helped me later in life to see it as part of my nature—a kind of check that keeps me striving, as well as a character flaw that keeps me from true success. I guess it's kind of okay to admit your flaws as long as it pushes you to defeat its losing ways at least 51% of the time. Wow. That's a whopper! Still, it's a difficult balancing act, navigating the sense of being both skilled and insufficient.

In my teens, I was still that small, thin kid who loved to play sports, who believed in his heart that he was destined for something great. But now, I was also someone who thought he understood the complexities of life (to a greater extent anyway).

Wrestling

In my sophomore year, I decided to expand my athletic horizons by joining the wrestling team. While I initially believed my karate training would provide a solid foundation, I quickly discovered that wrestling required a completely different set of skills.

I faced a significant personal challenge: managing my asthma. While I kept my condition to myself, it presented a constant obstacle that I had to manage. Keeping an inhaler nearby ready to use if I needed it. And also, learning to manage the attacks proactively, to mitigate the attacks as much as possible by using it therapeutically beforehand.

Wrestling emphasized takedowns, grappling, and pinning techniques, which were vastly different from the striking and blocking techniques I had used in karate. The close-quarters combat and physical intensity of wrestling presented a unique set of challenges.

Wrestling proved to be a grueling yet rewarding experience. Competing in the 115 weight division and moving up to the 135-pound weight class over three years, I was exposed to the intense world of competitive sports. The practices were physically demanding, often pushing me to my limits. However, they also instilled in me a mental toughness and discipline that would serve me well in my later martial arts training.

Despite the initial learning curve, I found wrestling to be incredibly rewarding. The intense practices and competitive matches forced me to reach beyond my comfort zone and develop a strong mental toughness. It also provided that team dynamic that doesn't develop the same way in karate, where the challenges are mostly as individuals.

While karate and wrestling may have seemed disparate at first, I eventually realized that they were actually complementary. The discipline and focus I had developed through karate proved invaluable in wrestling. Additionally, the strength and conditioning I had gained from martial arts training helped me to excel in the physically demanding sport of wrestling.

The weight classes in wrestling were strict, and maintaining my weight required a level of behavioral control that I hadn't experienced before. I had to be mindful of everything I ate and drank. Wrestling was as much about technique and strategy as it was about strength and endurance. Understanding how to leverage my weight, find angles, and exploit weaknesses in my opponents were lessons that I would carry forward into every other martial art I would practice.

As I progressed through the lighter weight classes, my natural speed and strength became increasingly apparent advantages. These physical attributes allowed me to dominate many of my opponents. However, I soon learned a valuable lesson: while physical prowess can be a significant asset, it is by no means the sole determinant of success.

Technique, it turned out, was the true equalizer. I observed firsthand as our coach demonstrated these techniques during practice. By paying close attention to his every move, I began to understand the nuances of each technique. I learned to anticipate my opponent's actions and to respond with precise countermoves. The more I practiced, the more ingrained these techniques became.

This realization shifted my perspective. I understood that while physical attributes could give me an edge, it was technical mastery that would truly set me apart. By honing my skills and developing a deep understanding of the sport, I was able to elevate my performance.

Track

Joining the track team in my sophomore year was a decision driven by my desire to stay active and challenge myself after the wrestling season ended, even though I knew my physical attributes might not align perfectly with the typical track and field events. Being a short guy, I was pretty fast for my height, but I was never going to match the speed of the taller, more athletic jocks who dominated the sprints. My coaches recognized this, so I was pointed towards the 330 low hurdles and high jump (also, not a short-guy event). These were among the least popular events and I was needed to have someone in the competition.

The high hurdles, with their height, were clearly designed for those with longer legs, and high jump was similarly more suited for taller athletes. But I was determined to make the most of what I had.

At the junior varsity level, I found my niche in the 330 low hurdles, where I was fast enough to be competitive and even placed a few times. That sense of accomplishment, despite not being the fastest overall, was a reward in itself.

As a high jumper, I managed to achieve a personal milestone by clearing a height equal to my own, which felt like a significant achievement. Although it wasn't enough to propel me to the varsity level, it was a challenge to my will and determination. There came a time however when I looked at all the varsity high-jumpers and noticed that all of them were much taller than I was. If they could accomplish what I had, the ability to jump their height, they would be starting way above what I could hope to achieve.

Since I couldn't dunk a basketball, there was really no hope in being anything more than a JV high jumper.

One of the things I really did enjoy was being pulled into the mile-relay team. I was pulled in to be with the other JV sprinters who were all football players as well. So I got in pretty good with some of the jocks. I ran the third leg—the slowest leg. Despite this, our team performed well and competed with heart.

Participating in track also had the unexpected benefit of helping me manage my asthma. Running regularly and pushing myself in the 330 low hurdles and mile relay required me to build stamina and learn how to control my breathing, which was crucial for an asthma sufferer. The consistent physical activity improved my overall lung capacity and endurance.

I became more attuned to recognizing the early signs of an asthma attack and learned techniques to manage my breathing more effectively. Track practice, with its rigorous workouts and need for sustained effort, became a practical way to strengthen my respiratory system and manage my condition, turning what could have been a limiting factor into an opportunity for personal growth and resilience.

Reflecting on my time on the track team, I realize that perhaps I could have found greater success in a sport that better suited my physical attributes. My compact stature and quickness, while advantageous in certain sport, were not ideal for the longer distances and sustained speed required for track and field. While I managed to find some success on the junior varsity level, the competitive nature of varsity proved to be a significant challenge. Listening to my own narrative about my experiences in track truly reveals the imposter within. But, looking back 40 years later, I'm wondering if it was all a wasted effort.

Despite these constraints, I don't view my time on the track team as a waste. It was a valuable experience that taught me a great deal about myself and my body. I formed friendships with my teammates, and the rigorous training regimen helped me develop endurance and perseverance.

In the end, the most important lesson I learned was the value of self-awareness. Recognizing my physical limitations allowed me to redirect my focus and pursue other avenues where I could excel.

Senior Year

By my senior year, my focus had shifted. I chose to concentrate on boxing and preparing for my upcoming black belt test, which meant stepping away from track and wrestling.

My high school years were a strange paradox. On the surface, I was a model student. I could effortlessly absorb information, ace tests, and finish assignments with ease.

My classmates often marveled at my academic prowess, and teachers praised my ability to grasp complex concepts. But beneath this facade of academic success, I struggled with a profound lack of identity. I was a cool guy, a smart guy, a karate guy, a conceited guy; I was all these and also an imposter.

The problem was that my intelligence sometimes felt like a burden rather than a blessing. My ability to coast through coursework without much effort made me feel disconnected from my peers. It was as if I were a spectator, observing the struggles of others while effortlessly gliding past them. This detachment, combined with a certain laziness, led to a lack of motivation and a sense of apathy.

It also became a weakness in follow through, which hinted at a quandary I would struggle with all my life.

When something comes easily, it becomes easy to be satisfied with mediocrity; it's easy to be good but not so easy to be great.

This philosophy clearly held me back from being that truly top-tier student. Instead of striving for the Ivy League, I was satisfied with Junior College. Quite frankly, I'll never know what greater levels of success I might have found. Years later I would learn more about this failure to execute haunting my personality.

My academic achievements, while impressive, were also a source of frustration. I often found myself rushing through tests, eager to finish as quickly as possible. I was more concerned about being first to finish, knowing I should go back and double-check my work.

I'm forced to wonder if I was just going fast just to show off? If the answer is yes, then I'm sure I would have got some answers wrong in my haste.

This haste sometimes led to careless mistakes, which I would later regret. Despite this careless philosophy, I still managed to achieve high grades, almost without trying. It was as if I had a built-in cheat code that allowed me to bypass the challenges faced by my less gifted classmates.

As I write this I am forced to wonder if the term gifted was both a blessing and a curse. Once labeled this way, it set an expectation for success and cast a negative shadow over any struggle.

I developed a less than ideal attitude that if I could get a B with no effort, then I wouldn't try for an A. So in the end, my 3.72 GPA was only a top 30 of my graduating class.

This ease of success, however, was a double-edged sword. It prevented me from reaching my full potential and ultimately hindered my college aspirations. While my parents encouraged us to pursue higher education and offered to pay for tuition, I was too lazy and ignorant to take the necessary steps. I missed the deadlines for applying to four-year universities and, as a result, found myself settling for community college.

The shining light through this reality is that is where I would meet my future wife. Had I gone directly to a four-year university, we likely would never have met.

Through the years, I continued to teach, train, and move up the ranks in our karate system. The requirements for promotion in our dojo were based on a combination of dedication, and commitment. It requires consistent practice, regular attendance, and a willingness to push oneself and others to the limits. I found this system to be both rewarding and demanding. There was no additional testing for second degree or beyond—the time teaching and training is the test.

Further commitment is demonstrated through this dedication. Once an instructor has more than one black belt student, then those who stick around become the ranking belts. Those who don't stop where they're at. The challenge is inherently addressed through time on the mat.

As I progressed through the ranks, I began to take on more responsibilities within the dojo. I assisted Sensei Rosas in teaching classes, helped with administrative tasks, helped organize and warm up the competition teams. For several sessions, Sensei Rosas moved to night-shift and asked me to take over classes for most of the year. These experiences not only enhanced my organizational skills but also developed my motivational skills, leadership abilities and sense of community.

Once I had the experience of leading a class on my own, from the beginning, I knew it was only time that would dictate my opportunity to open my own school.

The balance between my academic and martial arts pursuits was often precarious. There were times when the demands of one seemed to overshadow the other. But through it all, I managed to maintain a reasonable level of success in both areas. My experiences in high school taught me the importance of finding a healthy balance between work and play, between intellectual pursuits and personal passions.

Another challenge I faced was the realization that my "Gifted Classes" in junior high had not adequately prepared me for the rigor of high school English. I found myself struggling to write coherent paragraphs and essays, which significantly impacted my performance in English composition courses.

Determined to improve my writing skills, I dedicated myself to becoming a more avid reader. I expanded my viewpoint by seeking new genres, from classic literature to contemporary fiction, instead of martial arts magazines and book. By immersing myself in different writing styles and perspectives, I was able to develop a better understanding of grammar, syntax, and vocabulary.

Having required reading in my Literature classes forced me to engage. Brave New World, The Catcher in the Rye and Animal Farm had their impact on my intellect and psyche.

Over the course of my sophomore year, I made significant strides in my writing skills. My essays became more focused, well-organized, and coherent. I was proud of the progress I had made and the confidence I had gained. It was a goal I had set for myself and within one semester had shown marked improvement.

Despite the challenges of being a minority in a new environment, I was often perceived as one of the "smart ones." This stereotype, while flattering, also placed additional pressure on me to excel academically. It was a paradox and a conundrum, as it both highlighted my abilities and reinforced the idea that I had to meet certain expectations to fit in.

I wasn't always the student who sat in the front of the class, but at some point, something clicked. I realized that if I placed myself where the action was—right in front of the teacher—I could shape how they perceived me. I began moving toward the front row in every class, making sure I was visible and ready to engage.

Copyright © 2025 Darryl Vidal

Sitting up there gave me a sense of control, and it wasn't long before I noticed the subtle advantages. Teachers seemed to pay more attention to the students who appeared eager and involved, and I made it a point to be one of them.

I was no longer the quiet, and smart Asian kid in the back of the class. I became the vocal, obnoxious, know-it-all, wannabe teacher's pet in front of the class. From my perch up front I could interrupt the teacher and then look back at my classmates for effect. It was a new behavior nexus. One that required a bit of narcissism to execute.

My approach wasn't just about proximity; it was about participation. I started becoming a vocal part of every class discussion. Whenever a question was thrown out, my hand was one of the first to shoot up. Even when I wasn't entirely sure of the answer, I spoke up with confidence.

Over time, I noticed that the more I participated, the more teachers began to see me as a serious, engaged student. I figured if they liked me, they'd be more likely to cut me some slack if things got dicey, whether it was about grades or disciplinary issues.

Copyright © 2025 Darryl Vidal

Which I also learned to take advantage of. Being tardy no longer was a concern. Although I didn't arrive late on purpose, some teachers were more lenient, especially toward the star pupil.

This strategy worked on a deeper level too. By sitting in the front and being active in class, I started to feel more connected to the material. It was like I had positioned myself for success, both socially and academically. Teachers responded well to my enthusiasm, and I felt like I had a small edge when it came to navigating the ups and downs of school life.

While I never could achieve a perfect 4.0, I consistently earned A's and B's, demonstrating my commitment to learning and growth.

In my Government class, I had an unexpected test situation that could've gone sideways, but instead, it turned into a moment that cemented my strategy of staying on the teacher's good side. I had to miss a test because of a sick day, and when I returned to class, I wasn't sure how Mr. Garner, the teacher, would handle it. He was a no-nonsense guy, but he had a reputation for being fair. When I explained the situation, he said, "Okay, let's see what you've got," and proceeded to make an impromptu performance out of my makeup test.

Without warning, Mr. Garner grabbed the test sheet and started firing off the questions at breakneck speed, barely giving me time to breathe between them. He didn't slow down for a second, rattling off question after question, each one faster than the last. But I had been paying attention all semester, so I rattled off the answers just as quickly, without hesitation. I didn't need to stop and think—I knew the material—cold. Question after question, I nailed each one, and by the time we were done, Mr. Garner nodded, impressed. "That's an A," he said, loud enough for the whole class to hear.

But it wasn't just about the grade. I realized later that it was a bit of a show—one Mr. Garner enjoyed putting on. He was using me as an example for the rest of the class, showcasing the benefits of being an engaged student. It was his way of saying, "This is what happens when you pay attention." And while I appreciated the A, I knew it wasn't just about acing the test; it was about the relationship I had built with Mr. Garner through my participation and dedication in class. Sitting up front and being vocal had paid off once again.

A more foreboding example that would haunt me for the future was when I told him I didn't know where I was going to college, that I was considering starting at Chaffey Junior College.

He was dumbfounded. "What? Why? You should be applying to UCLA, or at least Cal Poly (Pomona)."

I didn't know how to respond. I just stood there.

Then in the next minute another student came forward and said they were going to enroll in Chaffey Junior College. He said, "That's a good choice." His tone was different even knowing that I was sitting right in front of their discussion.

I later asked him why he said I should seek out a university based on the discussion I had just witnessed. He said, "Because with your grades and intellect, you should be going directly to the university. Most students that go to JC quit and never go back."

This stung. Was I short-changing my opportunities? Was the lazy Darryl not doing good enough for the talented Darryl? I vowed that I would complete junior college and then surely move on to a University. I refused to become one of his statistics.

Junior College to University

As I transitioned from high school to college, I wasn't well-prepared to take on new challenges. As a gift for my 18th birthday, my Auntie Baby (my father's wealthy sister), bought me plane tickets to spend the Summer in Manila. What a grand thoughtful present. Part of the idea was that she, being quite the socialite in Manila, would introduce me to some filmmakers and possibly get me into the movies in the Philippines. It ended up that I spent Summer hanging with my cousins living the life of a wealthy socialite at the center of things.

We partied and went to night clubs and hung out with friends. My aunt did line up a couple of meetings, but nothing really panned out. I'm still thankful for the thought and effort and developed lifelong relationships with my cousins.

Unfortunately, by the time I returned, school was almost ready to start and I had done nothing towards enrollment. So my buddy and I enrolled at Chaffey as a default. In fact, he even filled out the application for me. What a friend.

My first junior college years were a time of internal conflict and self-doubt. I was torn between my academic abilities and my lack of motivation. I felt like a misfit, a high-achiever who didn't apply to a university. It would take years for me to reconcile these conflicting aspects of my identity and discover my true path.

My decision to attend classes only two days a week was a strategic move to balance my academic pursuits with my passion for karate. While it may have seemed like an easy workload, it also presented its own set of challenges. The reduced class schedule meant that I had to be more disciplined and efficient with my study time. I had to learn to prioritize tasks, manage my time effectively, and stay focused on multiple work requirements simultaneously. I know, everyone has to do it.

After starting full-time at Hughes as Telecommunications Technician I completed my AA at Chaffey and followed through by enrolling at Cal State San

Copyright © 2025 Darryl Vidal

Bernardino the following Fall—Mr. Garner's words haunting me.

Those four years were a slog. I'd commute to Anaheim Hills in the morning and then make the trek to Cal State San Bernardino—48 miles or an hour and a half on the 91 and 15 freeway with the best traffic. On two other nights I was still teaching with Sensei Rosas in Chino.

Through this period between 1982 and 1988, six years, I would: move to Alta Loma with my parents, start junior college, play with the Turbos, still teaching karate twice a week and competing on the weekends. Not the busiest schedule of anyone ever, but medium to very busy.

Then in '83 I got hooked into the Karate Kid rehearsals in July, August, and filming in October with the final tournament scenes in December 1983. Got married in '86 so finally in 1988 I completed my Bachelor's Degree in Business Administration.

The commute from Alta Loma to Chino, while time-consuming, was a small price to pay for the opportunity to continue teaching karate under the guidance of Sensei Rosas. My involvement in the dojo provided a sense of purpose and fulfillment that I often lacked in my academic life. Teaching karate allowed me to share my knowledge and experience with others, while also challenging myself to become a better martial artist.

I yearned to deepen my connection to my native art form of Filipino Escrima. I made efforts to learn from experienced practitioners but there were no schools in the local area. All the well known escrima schools were in San Diego or Stockton. Undeterred, I sought out opportunities to train informally with local escrima practitioners and dedicated students.

A couple were Filipino martial artists I met at Hughes. We would train at lunch at a nearby park. Each knew a variety of drills and practice routines. Some similar, some not, but always something more to add to my skill set.

FMA is a unique martial art because the student starts with weaponry. The escrima sticks are employed like extensions of the hands and less like a club or bat. The rattan sticks are more dense than bamboo but lighter than oak or other solid wood. The stick is more intended for traumatizing the flesh or joints than knocking an opponent out.

Unlike karate, FMA focuses less on form and derives its lethality from flow and momentum. The footwork of FMA is as intricate as boxing, utilizing oblique and triangular stepping in concert with the circular flow of the sticks.

You might think that this bamboo-like stick is harmless until I smash your knuckles and hammer your joints with them.

Once the student becomes adept at single- and double-stick drills and sparring, bladed weapons are introduced, with knives being at the core of the Escrimadors concealed weaponry. Though most men carry a folding knife in their pocket or on their belt, people are surprised to discover that my everyday carry (EDC) knife is a 9" fixed blade tactical knife on my left hip (because I'm carrying a gun on my right hip). And I can draw it and switch hands faster than you can draw yours from your pocket.

I joke with my students that I may not knock you out with the stick but I will turn your face into a bloody pulp. After I'm done you'll wish I knocked you out! Because of the light weight of the stick, I can hit the opponent multiple times in the time it would take to swing a bat or bo staff.

From there, the FMA student moves to empty hand fighting, transitioning the flowing movements of the stick and blade to the empty hand, in a devastating fusillade of high speed striking methods not dissimilar to boxing and Wing Chun.

One of the most valuable aspects of my training was the opportunity to learn from experienced practitioners. While I didn't have the benefit of formal classes, I was fortunate to receive guidance from a few assistant instructors who I met in different settings and generously shared their knowledge and expertise.

As I progressed in my FMA training, I began to blend the various practice drills and patterns into a more cohesive system. I focused on fluid transitions, variations, and real-world applications. My goal was to develop a well-rounded and effective FMA-based fighting style based on the diverse systems I studied.

Through my dedication to escrima, I discovered a deeper connection to my Filipino heritage. The martial art became a channel for me to express my cultural identity and celebrate my roots. It was a way to honor my ancestors and connect with the rich history of the Philippines.

Escrima derives its power from momentum and flow. It's quite a departure from the methods taught in karate. This focus on mechanics also taught me valuable life lessons, such as resilience and adaptability. The flow and footwork of FMA is a stark departure from karate—so much so that I don't encourage beginning karate students to cross-train in FMA.

As I continued to practice escrima, I felt a growing sense of pride and belonging. I was no longer just a Filipino American; I was a Filipino warrior. But alas, the spectre of the imposter weighed heavy on my cultural being. I mean, I didn't even speak the language and could document no lineage for my escrima.

The Turbos

It all started with a spark of creativity, the simplest of chords, and a couple of buddies with a shared love of music and martial arts. We called ourselves The Turbos, a name that was equal parts homage to my favorite car, the Porsche 911 Turbo and a nod to the era's fascination with all things fast and cool. The band was born in the most organic way possible: just a few high school buddies who enjoyed jamming together.

I played bass because Tim played guitar and we didn't need another guitar player if we didn't have a bass player. I recruited my older brother Irwin, despite his protests, he sat in as our drummer. Irwin always insisted he was doing it as a favor to us—helping out little brother and his friends—but made it clear that he didn't see himself as our permanent drummer. "I've got other things going on," he would say, his tone casual but his talent undeniable.

For me, the musical dalliance began with the most basic building blocks—the barre chords that Irwin had taught me just a few months earlier. As I practiced, I found myself piecing together simple but catchy tunes. I wrote a handful of overly simplistic songs, the kind of lyrics and melodies that only a teenager with his first guitar could dream up. Two of the earliest were "I May be Missing" and "I'm Too Cool For You!"—neither of which would win any songwriting awards, but they were fun, upbeat, and surprisingly well-received by our friends. Despite their

Copyright © 2025 Darryl Vidal

simplicity, these songs were the foundation of what would soon become a real band. In our minds anyway.

Of course, we also threw in a couple of cover songs to round out our set. Our renditions of Twist and Shout and La Bamba were always crowd-pleasers, though I'll be the first to admit that my bass playing was still rough around the edges. I wasn't a technically skilled musician, but I made up for it with enthusiasm and rhythm.

At first, it was all about having fun—just jamming in the garage and playing for anyone willing to listen. But something shifted once we realized that people were genuinely into what we were doing. Our friends, mostly from high school and martial arts class, started asking us to play at house parties, and before long, we had our first real gigs. It was a surreal experience.

We were just a bunch of teenagers with borrowed instruments and a classic Ludwig drum kit, yet we were getting asked to play in front of crowds. The house parties were a riot. Packed living rooms and garages turned into makeshift concert halls, and we'd blast through our setlist of original songs with all the swagger of a group that thought they were already rock stars.

The funny thing was, as much as Irwin insisted he wasn't really part of the band, his drumming was a crucial part of our sound. He had an effortless rhythm, and every time we played, he elevated our music. It was clear we needed him, even if he pretended otherwise. It wasn't long before we outgrew the high school parties and started playing for bigger audiences. I still remember the rush of getting paid for the first time. It wasn't much—just enough to cover gas money and fast food—but it felt like validation. We were a real "professional" band.

In our second paying gig, we were able to rent our own PA system, instead of running our vocals through a spare guitar amp or even my own bass amp sometimes.

As The Turbos began to evolve and gain more attention, it became clear that we needed a permanent drummer. Irwin, though incredibly talented, would always say, "even if you make it big, I don't want to be your drummer." As much as we loved having him behind the drum kit, we knew he was not really into it. So, after a series of gigs, we started looking for someone who could step into that role for the long haul.

That's when Robbie, one of Tim's high school friends, entered the picture. Robbie had been a part of his extended social circle for years and had always shown an interest in our band. When we asked him to sit in for a few practices, he was ready for us. He offered to let us use his garage, which was the clincher. Not only would his parents let us use the garage, but we could leave the equipment there, which is huge—if not a bit self-serving.

When we auditioned Robbie for the Turbos, I was a bit skeptical. We had specific beats in mind for our songs, and I wasn't sure if he could keep up with the tight, driving rhythms that our sound depended on. But as soon as he sat behind the kit and started playing, it became clear that he had a natural feel for rock beats.

Robbie picked up on the basic rhythms almost immediately, locking into the pulse of each song without needing much guidance. It was refreshing to see someone jump into the groove so seamlessly, and it gave the whole band a sense of confidence in his ability.

What really set Robbie apart was his energy and enthusiasm, especially compared to Irwin. Robbie genuinely liked our music, and it showed—he played with a fire that Irwin never quite managed to bring. It was refreshing. I no longer had to convince my brother to come along, or that we'd pay for the beer. Actually, we made RobCat pay for the beer.

The rest of us fed off his intensity, and rehearsals started to feel more alive and full of potential. Robbie didn't just hit the beats; he added a level of passion that brought out the best in our songs. In those first few rehearsals, it was clear he was the perfect fit for the Turbos.

Unlike Irwin, who saw drumming for the Turbos as a temporary gig, Robbie fully embraced becoming a Turbo. He brought a fresh energy to the band, and suddenly, we felt like we had a complete lineup. Robbie wasn't just filling a role—he became a core member of The Turbos, and with him on drums, we started to gel more as a band. We dubbed him RobCat.

With RobCat, we found stability. He wasn't Irwin, but he didn't have to be. Robbie had his own style, a more laid-back approach that worked well with our growing sound. He was a year younger than us, so, less mature in a good way.

He quickly became as passionate about the band as we were, attending every practice, every gig, and adding his own flair to our original songs. He became a true Turbo, and as we continued playing and recording, it felt like we had found our groove.

Soon, our reputation started spreading beyond the typical high school crowd. One of the strangest and most unexpected developments in The Turbos' brief career was landing gigs at middle schools. These weren't your typical audiences, but for whatever reason, the students went absolutely wild for us.

Since Tim volunteered at a couple of the middle schools in the area, he had the connections to get us booked for their afternoon entertainment sessions. It was a unique opportunity, as we hadn't played for a younger crowd before, and these school gigs allowed us to refine our set in front of an audience that was full of energy and curiosity. Tim's connections made the scheduling easy, and the school staff appreciated having something fresh and fun for the students.

These performances became a great way for us to grow our stage presence and learn how to engage a crowd that wasn't just there for a typical rock show. The kids' excitement was contagious, and playing for them added a new level of energy to our music. It was rewarding to see how much they enjoyed the performance, and it also helped us build a local reputation that gave us a stronger foothold in the community.

I still remember stepping onto the stage at one of these schools, expecting polite applause and maybe a few shouts. Instead, the kids erupted into cheers, as if we were the next big thing. We felt like The Beatles—well, maybe a local version of them. The energy in the room was electric, and these young crowds treated us like rock gods, singing along to our original songs as if they had known them for years.

At one middle school gig, a group of kids rushed the stage during I'm Too Cool For You!, dancing and jumping along to the music and falling over the amps. It was such a surreal moment. Our original songs, which I had always thought of as rough, juvenile attempts at music, were somehow connecting with these audiences in a way we hadn't anticipated. The adrenaline rush of those performances was unlike anything else. We may have been a small, local band, but those days, we felt invincible.

One of the most exciting, yet ultimately disappointing, moments in The Turbos story came when we nearly landed a gig to open for the legendary Oingo Boingo. It all started when we heard that a local radio station was holding a contest for bands to open at a major show. We thought, "Why not?" So, we submitted a tape of our best songs and waited for what felt like an eternity. Amazingly, we made it to the final selection round, competing against another up-and-coming local band, The Untouchables. We could already picture ourselves up on stage, playing to thousands of fans, sharing the stage with Oingo Boingo.

But as fate would have it, we lost the gig to The Untouchables. We were crushed. In our minds, this was our big break, and it had slipped through our fingers. But looking back, that near miss was just another crazy chapter in the story of our band. It pushed us to keep going, even if we weren't destined to play alongside our musical heroes. The disappointment turned into motivation.

Recording Our First Tracks

As The Turbos began picking up steam and landing more paid gigs, we knew that the next step was to elevate our sound. Tim, Robbie, and I were solid in our own right, but there was something missing—someone who could bring a real artistic dimension to the band and take us to the next level. That's when we connected with JL, a super-talented singer and musician who would completely change the dynamic of The Turbos.

JL was unlike anyone we had ever played with before. He was a true multi-talented artist, with a voice that could shift effortlessly between the tones of Billy Joel and the melodic power of Elton John or the smooth croon of Paul McCartney. He wasn't just a singer, though; JL could play just about anything. His musical repertoire was staggering—he could perform hundreds of the most popular songs from memory, and he did so with an effortless confidence that captivated anyone who listened. When he joined us, it felt like we were finally a complete band.

Of course, compared to JL, we were way out of our league musically, but with him playing keyboards and some guitar, he redefined the Turbos. Funny thing was, he like our songs too!

With JL on board, we started to refine our sound, moving beyond our simple originals and adding covers of classics that we had never been able to tackle before. His voice became the centerpiece of our performances, and his ability to switch between keyboard and lead guitarist gave our music a versatility we hadn't known we were capable of.

JL didn't just fill a role—he made The Turbos a real thing. He brought a level of artistry and musicality that turned us from a high school band into something that could hold its own in front of a paying audience. His ability to connect with a crowd, play flawlessly, and sing like a seasoned professional made every gig feel more serious, more real. With him, we weren't just a group of friends messing around; we were a band with real potential.

As The Turbos started to gain momentum, we decided it was time to get serious about recording. With some of the money we had earned from gigs, we booked a session at a professional studio to lay down our first tracks.

We heard about a guy who did band recordings. We met with him at lunch and he told us his studio was in his condo. But he had a garage converted to a sound studio. As it turned out, we used the garage and his bedroom which was converted so we could set up the amps and drums and play as a full band while he ran the 8-track recorder from the garage studio.

Copyright © 2025 Darryl Vidal

It wasn't pretty, but it was an 8-track recording with a sound engineer. That's a lot better than a boombox cassette recorder.

We recorded ten songs from our repertoire, most of which were original compositions that I had written. These tracks weren't sophisticated by any means—simple chord progressions and lyrics that didn't dive too deep—but they were ours. These were simplistic songs in the vein of "I want to hold your Hand" and "I Saw Her Standing There."

The fact that we were creating something from scratch made every recording session feel monumental. Recording in a studio taught me a lot. It forced us to refine our sound and think about music in a more professional way. Suddenly, we weren't just playing to fill the air at parties or schools—we were creating something lasting, something that could be played back and judged long after we'd left the studio. I realized just how much work went into making a polished track. There were multiple takes, long hours, and plenty of frustration, but at the end of the day, hearing our songs come to life in that polished, professional format was worth it.

The transition from the humble 8-track home studio to the professional Wine Tree Studios in Claremont was a significant milestone in our musical evolution. The 24-track capabilities of the studio offered a level of flexibility and precision that we had never before experienced.

By breaking up the recording sessions into multiple sessions, we were able to bring in additional musicians and experiment with different sounds. The added flexibility allowed us to create a more dynamic and layered sound for our music.

Instead of trying to do 4 songs in an 8-hour session. We booked multiple sessions for each song. The difference between the 8-track songs and the 24-track songs was immediately apparent. The increased track count enabled us to achieve a richer, more complex soundscape. We were able to add subtle nuances and harmonies that were simply impossible with our previous setup.

A Life-Changing Party

One of the wildest parts of being in The Turbos was the unpredictable nature of the house parties we played. It was at one of these raucous parties, packed with teenagers dancing, drinking, and having the time of their lives, that I first crossed paths with someone who would later become incredibly important to me—my future wife. Of course, I didn't know it at the time. She was just another face in the crowd, enjoying the music and the atmosphere. But that moment, amidst the chaos of a typical Turbos party, marked the beginning of something that would shape the rest of my life.

Other party shenanigans were legendary. One memorable incident took place at a local dairy farm, of all places. What started as an ordinary gathering quickly spiraled into chaos when some of the sheep managed to break loose. In a scene straight out of a comedy, the animals ran wild, knocking over equipment and sending everyone into a frenzied attempt to regain control. We couldn't help but laugh as the party transformed into an impromptu rodeo, with guests chasing sheep through the fields. It was the kind of bizarre moment that stayed with you, more hilarious in hindsight than it was at the time.

Not all parties had such lighthearted endings, though. There was one tragic night when a close-knit group of friends found themselves in a violent altercation with local gang members. What started as a regular party escalated into a nightmare as tensions flared. The fight ended in bloodshed, with several friends getting stabbed. Thankfully, no one died, but in the immediate aftermath, we were left in the dark, unsure of who had survived and what had truly transpired. For days, the uncertainty gnawed at us, as rumors and conflicting stories swirled through our circles, each more terrifying than the last.

The emotional weight of that night lingered for a long time. It was a reminder that the wild nights we once considered carefree could turn dangerous without warning. It made us all more aware of how fragile our sense of invincibility really was.

When I look back on the time I spent with The Turbos, it feels like a wild, fast-paced ride. What started as a casual project between friends had turned into something real—a band that played gigs, recorded songs, and almost hit the big time. We weren't just jamming in garages anymore; we were performing for actual audiences, and people were enjoying what we had created. There were plenty of highs and lows, but each experience taught me something valuable.

While my brothers had their natural, almost effortless musical talents, being part of The Turbos helped me discover my own hidden abilities. It wasn't the technical skills that set me apart, but rather my rhythm, my ability to create something with heart, and my drive to keep pushing forward, even when things didn't always go as planned. Being in the band opened my eyes to the possibilities of music and what could happen when passion, creativity, and a bit of luck collided.

The story of The Turbos may have been brief, but it was unforgettable. It was a chapter of my life filled with music, friendship, and unexpected opportunities. Though we never became rock stars, we had our moment in the sun, and for a bunch of high school friends, that was more than enough.

The Turbos recordings are still in the archives. I'm still reminded to play them for my wife and kids every now and then with the regular response being, "These are great, we should release them." But I think their time has come and gone.

Early Training & Influences

Kung Fu Movie Night

In the early 1970s, my introduction to martial arts came in the form of kung-fu movies that my brothers and I couldn't get enough of. Every weekend, we'd gather around the TV to watch these larger-than-life films, captivated by the fluid movements, the power, and the mysticism that seemed to surround the martial artists. The heroes in those movies were untouchable—effortlessly dispatching waves of enemies with precision and grace. Watching them charged us up like crazy. The moment the credits rolled, we were ready to spring into action, our imaginations running wild with the possibilities of what we could do ourselves.

As soon as the movie ended, we'd head straight outside, energized and inspired to recreate the epic battles we had just witnessed. We didn't have any formal training, but that didn't stop us from throwing punches, kicks, and spinning around like we were in the middle of our own kung-fu movie. What we lacked in technique, we made up for in enthusiasm. Our "fights" were more like improvised dance routines than choreographed sequences, full of wild movements and made-up rules. It wasn't about winning or losing—it was about trying to capture that feeling of being unstoppable, just like the heroes on the screen.

It was something every Asian American kid could connect with. Baseball, football and basketball, although fun and popular with our neighborhood friends, we actually

Copyright © 2025 Darryl Vidal

looked like the people in these films, and the white kids didn't, and couldn't. It was a thing.

We were so into kung-fu movies that when The Chinese Connection came to theaters, it was a big event for us. My parents knew how much my brothers and I loved martial arts films, so they took us to the drive-in to see it, along with Five Fingers of Death as the double feature. I still remember the excitement of piling into the car, knowing we were about to witness something epic.

At the drive-in, we were glued to the screen as Bruce Lee exploded onto the scene with his iconic intensity and lightning-fast movements. Watching those films under the stars with my family felt like we were part of something bigger, like the energy of the kung-fu world we admired so much was alive around us. By the time the movies ended, we were buzzing with adrenaline, ready to try out everything we'd just seen. Those drive-in nights, especially seeing Bruce Lee in action, were unforgettable and only deepened our obsession with martial arts.

Even as I immersed myself in martial arts movies, a sense of imposter syndrome quietly crept in. As much as I idolized the characters on screen, I couldn't shake the feeling that I didn't truly belong in the world they represented. The heroes in those films—whether Bruce Lee in The Chinese Connection or the masters in Five Fingers of Death—were almost always Chinese or Japanese. Martial arts at the time, at least in the public eye, were so closely tied to these cultures that it felt like there wasn't space for someone like me, a Filipino-American kid, to fully claim that world as my own.

That twang of doubt hit me hardest during those moments when I tried to picture myself as one of those heroes. I could mimic the moves, throw punches and kicks just like them, but I didn't look like them, and I wasn't from the same cultural background. It made me question whether I had a right to pursue martial arts so seriously.

First Karate Instructor

When we were still living in San Diego, my eldest brother took the first step that would set us all on the path to martial arts. He had discovered a local karate instructor, Mr. George Mique, who taught out of a humble garage dojo. There was no fancy signage or commercial studio, just a small group of students gathering in a quiet neighborhood. But what Mr. Mique lacked in formality, he made up for, with passion and tradition. His approach was simple—a structured introduction to the basics of karate, taught with a steady hand and a sharp focus on fundamentals.

After every lesson, my brother would come home buzzing with excitement. He was learning the foundational stances, the basic kicks, and punches—the essential building blocks of any karate practice. We'd see him practicing in the backyard, perfecting his horse stance or drilling his sidekicks against an invisible opponent. My middle brother and I couldn't help but watch in awe as he went through his routines, moving with a purpose we hadn't seen before.

My eldest brother became our first karate instructor. After his sessions with Mr. Mique, he'd gather us together and run through what he had learned that day. We'd mimic his movements, sometimes awkwardly at first, trying to get our bodies to move in ways that felt both familiar and foreign. Karate wasn't just about throwing punches—it was about precision, balance, and control, things that took time to develop. I can remember feeling like this stance stuff was a waste of time. I wanted to get directly into kicking and punching. The philosophy of development and mastery over time was lost on me at this age.

But my brother was patient. He broke down the stances for us, showing us how to root ourselves firmly to the ground, how to position our hands, and how to snap a punch with speed and power.

Our backyard became an extension of Mr. Mique's garage dojo. We practiced diligently, trying to mirror the techniques our brother passed down to us. At that age, there was something special about learning from him—it felt like we were being initiated into a secret world, one that only a select few could access. In some ways, our sessions in the backyard were even more intense than those in a formal dojo because there was no strict timetable, no boundaries to how long we could practice.

It's clear that those early lessons were more than just physical training. They taught us about balance, practice, building muscle memory and the importance of passing down knowledge. The need for instant gratification was tempered by our own lack of experience and coordination.

Vince didn't hoard what he learned—he shared it with us, and in doing so, he planted the seeds for what would become a lifelong journey in martial arts.

Now, we were building real skills, training in a way that connected us to something deeper. Even though we were young, we knew we were on to something special.

When we moved to Chino, we knew nothing and no one. Once school started, Vince met a friend who lived around the corner who was exposed to a lot of martial arts at an early age named Carlos. Even though he had the equipment and stories, I never saw him wearing a gi or claiming a belt rank. But his technique and fighting abilities were undeniable. He could move like a martial artist and had a ton of books to peruse when we weren't training. This was my first encounter with Bruce Lee's Fighting Methods, and his Tao of Jeet Kune Do.

He had a heavy bag hung in his garage by his dad who used to box. There we learned to kick into the bag. Round kicks, side kicks and back spins. All fundamental kicks in almost all martial arts.

Since he was open to teaching and we were ready to train, he started teaching us some basic Kung Fu moves. He wasn't a master, or even a Sensei, but he knew enough to give us a taste of real martial arts training. He also had some basic Escrima. Looking back, it was only the most rudimentary drills, but it was the first I was to see how fast and effective the flow of FMA could be.

Those lessons were an exciting new chapter, as they added a level of structure to the chaotic energy we had been channeling from the movies. Suddenly, our punches and kicks had form, and we began learning the fundamentals of power, balance, and focus. It felt like we were stepping into the world we had only seen in those films, but now we had the tools to back it up.

But despite all the time I spent practicing moves and mimicking what I saw in kung-fu movies and our new friend, there was one thing I still didn't have—a belt. I could throw punches and kicks with the best of them in my neighborhood, and I had even learned some techniques from neighbors of friends, but none of that came with an official rank.

A belt symbolized legitimacy in the martial arts world, a way of proving that your skills were recognized and that you had been trained in a structured way. Without one, I still felt like I was playing martial arts rather than truly being part of it.

I knew that if I wanted to be taken seriously, if I wanted to feel like a real martial artist, I needed more than just the informal training I had picked up along the way. I needed to walk into a proper karate studio, bow at the mat, and commit to a program that would guide me through the ranks. Earning a belt wasn't just about wearing a piece of colored fabric—it was about the practice, focus, and formal education that came with it. It was the one thing standing between me and the validation I craved.

I needed to prove to myself that I could make it through the rigorous structure of real karate training, not just what I'd picked up in backyards or from watching films. So, I decided it was time to make it official. I needed to step into a studio and earn my rank, starting from the ground up like everyone else. The belt was more than just a goal—it was the key to unlocking my full potential as a martial artist.

Those early experiences—both the movies and the backyard brawls—sparked a fire in me that would only grow over time. Martial arts became more than just something fun to do after watching a movie; it became a passion, something I knew I wanted to keep exploring as I grew older. And even in those early days, I could feel that martial arts wasn't just about fighting—it was about self-discovery and pushing the limits of what I could do physically and mentally.

This feeling didn't stop me from practicing or from being passionate about martial arts, but it was always there, lingering in the back of my mind. I wanted so badly to belong to this world that I admired, yet at times, it felt as if there was an invisible barrier between me and the authenticity of it all. Martial arts were so powerfully linked to specific Asian identities, and while I was 100% Filipino, I didn't see that same representation in the movies or in the martial arts community at large. It was like a subtle reminder that, despite my enthusiasm and dedication, I was somehow on the fringes of the very thing I loved.

Nunchucks

Our growing fascination with martial arts naturally led us to explore some of the most iconic weapons associated with martial arts and the nunchucks quickly captured our imagination. After watching Bruce Lee wield nunchucks with astonishing skill in The Chinese Connection and later in Enter the Dragon, we were hooked. His mastery of the weapon seemed almost magical, and we were eager to experience that same sense of power and fluidity. Inspired by Lee's performances, we decided to craft our own nunchucks, eager to try them out and see if we could replicate some of the impressive moves we had seen.

Initially, we made do with whatever materials we could find around the house. Our first attempts were clunky and rudimentary—using broom sticks, old table legs or pool cue ends connected by lengths of chain we cut from bike locks.

Later a trip to the hardware store found that screw eyes and short lengths of chain didn't cost much, which made for much more menacing nunchucks. These homemade nunchucks were heavy, noisy and cumbersome, and swinging them around often led to bruises and mishaps.

The good thing about learning and practicing nunchucks as a child is you get all the pain and injuries out of the way. When you pick them up as an adult, you already know what moves bring the most mistakes and pain—what moves to try and which moves to avoid at all costs.

Along with the bruised elbows and head shots, we also had the typical screw come loose and sling a single chuck into whatever got in the way, be it a mirror or best buddy.

We finally learned how to use rope which was 100% better than chain. Not only was it easier to make, it was quiet and light. It also didn't cause irreparable damage to an innocent bystander. However, our perseverance paid off as we learned more about the mechanics of the weapon.

Eventually, we upgraded to making nunchucks out of PVC pipe, which proved to be a game changer. The lighter material allowed for much faster, more controlled movements and reduced the risk of injury. This shift not only improved our technique but also made practicing with the nunchucks a lot more enjoyable. Our homemade weapons became a testament to our dedication and creativity, and they added a new dimension to our martial arts training, bringing us one step closer to the martial artists we aspired to be. Plus, the lighter plastic nunchucks proved to be the secret behind the speed of Bruce Lee's nunchaku demonstrations. In fact, in the Chinese Connection, you can see the nunchucks bending and flexing under the stress of the moves.

Escrima

The obscure martial art of the Philippines called escrima was barely known at the time, and the exposure we had was mostly informal and inconsequential.

We had seen it at the Faith Healer's house and Vince's friend in Chino had studied some with Dan Insosanto's school in Orange County. Almost any household with Filipino influence would include a wall display of the various weapons of the Philippines. It was so common, it only engendered a quick glance to acknowledge—this is a Filipino household.

It didn't even mean they studied the arts of Escrima, Kali or Arnis—the various names attributed to the FMA family of systems—but it surely left the impression that the Filipinos were warriors.

So throughout my life I would seek out various sources for FMA training. Was I just a kid trying to fit into something I could never truly be a part of? I was fascinated by the philosophy and the techniques, but I couldn't help feeling like an outsider looking in—like I was playing a role I wasn't born to fill.

I vowed that no matter what variety of systems I might study in my lifetime, my cultural connection to my

Copyright © 2025 Darryl Vidal

parent's homeland warranted its share of my attention—it would take years to fulfill. But I would fulfill it in the best way possible.

Karate Classes

At the age of 14, I discovered a world that would shape me in ways I never imagined—Kenpo Karate. It was the mid-1970s, and martial arts were not just a practice but a movement, riding high on the influence of Billy Jack, the first real American martial arts movie, Bruce Lee and kung fu movies that filled theater screens.

My introduction to Kenpo Karate came almost by chance when a friend from the neighborhood told me about classes being held at the Chino Parks and Recreation Department. Intrigued and eager for a real karate class, I signed up with Vinci.

We found ourselves under the tutelage of Instructor Joe Rosas. Joe wasn't your typical martial arts teacher running a big school. He had started small, teaching in his garage until the Parks and Rec program gave him an opportunity to share his knowledge with a larger audience. Joe was humble, but his dedication to his craft was apparent. His students respected him, and I remember being particularly impressed by two of his lead students, both women. One, Claudine Sill, would later become his first student to achieve the rank of black belt in November 1980—a milestone that inspired us all.

I recall Joe also had another senior student, someone who had trained under his instructor, Dan Guzman. This student had already reached the rank of black belt, setting an example of what dedication and commitment to Kenpo could lead to. For Vinci and me, this was a whole new world—one of discipline, hard work, and self-discovery.

Joe was more than just a karate instructor; he was a committed and caring mentor who genuinely invested in his students' well-being. One particular instance stands out vividly in my memory, showcasing his dedication and compassion.

At one point, when money was tight for my family, my oldest brother Vinci and I found ourselves in a difficult spot. We didn't have the $11 needed for the upcoming eight-week karate session, a modest amount that back then, represented a significant hurdle for us.

Knowing how much we valued our training, Joe didn't turn us away or suggest we find another way. Instead, he offered us a solution that spoke volumes about his character. He "hired" us to help with some work in his backyard. Joe was in the midst of having a retaining wall built and needed help moving bricks from one location to another.

For most of the day, Vinci and I labored under the hot sun, sweating profusely as we carried bricks two by two. It was grueling work, but Joe's offer meant that we could stay in class, and that was more important to us than anything else.

As I look back on that day, I sometimes wonder if there was an actual need to move all those bricks or if Joe had simply devised this task as a way to ensure we could continue our training.

Either way, his actions were a testament to his dedication and kindness. He found a way to keep us involved in karate, not just as students but as part of a community that cared for each other. Joe's generosity and resourcefulness allowed us to remain part of the dojo, reinforcing the sense of support and family that was at the heart of our martial arts journey.

I was always athletic. In my teens I could easily do 50 pushups and 15 pull ups. I was kid with boundless energy and a natural sense of rhythm. I played street baseball and football with my neighborhood friends, but Kenpo tapped into something deeper. It felt like unlocking a part of myself that had been waiting to be discovered. Kenpo Karate was not just about learning to fight; it was about mastering the art of movement, of timing, and precision.

From the very beginning, I was drawn to the acrobatic flair of kung fu. I had an innate flexibility and could kick with height and speed, performing techniques that seemed to defy gravity. The jumping, spinning, and flying kicks I had seen in the kung fu movies of Bruce Lee and later Jackie Chan became part of my daily practice, despite the fact that they weren't part of the standard Kenpo curriculum. In fact, my instructor never did high or flashy kicks. These weren't just stunts; they were expressions of what I was learning in the dojo—strength, balance, and control.

I also had a knack for simple gymnastics, which led me to master handstands, handsprings, and even some rough attempts at backflips. I began incorporating these skills into my martial arts training, using them to boost my strength and flexibility. The gymnastic moves added a dynamic edge to my practice, helping me become more agile and versatile in my martial arts techniques.

Instructor Joe Rosas noticed my potential, and I soon found myself advancing through the ranks faster than most of the other students. Within a year, I had earned my blue belt, a significant achievement for someone so new to the art. But I wasn't satisfied with that. I pushed myself even harder, and by December 1978, I had earned my green belt.

The Library Dojo

My passion for martial arts extended far beyond the hours spent in the dojo. Every week, I made it a point to visit the local library, where I would check out every book I could find on martial arts. I was particularly drawn to the writings of Fumio Demura, a renowned expert in traditional Japanese karate, whose books were both instructional and philosophical. Through Demura's writings, I learned that martial arts were as much about discipline and focus of the mind as the body. Little did I know that I would meet him a few years later.

Bruce Lee, of course, was the major influence. His book, Tao of Jeet Kune Do—the "Way of the Intercepting Fist"—challenged conventional ideas about martial arts. Lee's emphasis on fluidity, adaptability, and directness in combat fascinated me, and I began to incorporate his principles into my own training.

Then there was Mas Oyama, the founder of Kyokushin Karate, known for his incredible feats of strength and endurance. Reading about his system taught me that martial arts mastery required a lifetime of commitment.

Mas Oyama's "This is Karate" books were fundamentally different from the other martial arts books I had read. While many books focused on technique and kata, Oyama's approach was a raw, unapologetic look at the full potential of martial arts mastery, blending philosophy, power, and spectacle. He didn't just teach how to punch and kick—he showed the extremes of what the human body and mind could achieve.

Oyama famously broke bottles with his bare hands, fought and killed bulls, and demonstrated feats of strength that bordered on the mythical. This was where I first read about breaking rocks—something I found unbelievable at the time. It opened my eyes to the idea that martial arts were not just about self-defense or sport but about pushing the body and mind beyond perceived limits, into realms of near impossibility.

Books became my secondary dojo, where I could expand my understanding of martial arts beyond the physical techniques. They opened my mind to the philosophies and traditions behind the movements I was learning, connecting me to a history that stretched back centuries.

Kata & Kumite

By this time Joe started bringing a team of students to as many local karate tournaments as possible. Rosas Chino Kenpo Karate aka, RCKK, became a stalwart of Orange and Los Angeles county open karate tournaments of the late seventies and early eighties.

My first tournament as a blue belt was a memorable experience. I entered the competition focused solely on kumite, or sparring, and was thrilled to take first place. This victory was not just a personal achievement but also marked the beginning of a collection of trophies that would come to symbolize my achievements in martial arts.

After taking home the trophy for kumite, I vowed to do both kata and kumite divisions at the next tournament. Guess what happened, I took first place in both divisions, which started a streak of success where I would bring home at least two trophies, maybe not always first, but often enough.

Joe was never able to accumulate and account for the hundreds of trophies earned by his students during this era. Although he never once talked about it. For him, watching and leading his students was all he needed.

By the early 1980s, these competitions became a significant part of my martial arts experience, and I quickly found success in both kata and sparring divisions. Over the next few years, I amassed hundreds of trophies and awards, a testament to the dedication and hard work I put into my training.

We had a team of green and brown belts that would go and come home with a bevy of trophies that would make any dojo proud. Unfortunately for RCKK, being a parks and recreation dojo, we weren't able to display all these trophies in a dojo showcase.

I started to accumulate so many trophies that by the time we moved to Alta Loma, my dad built a trophy wall, by adding several wall shelves, to display all the trophies. In some cases, where they would have grand champions divisions, I might actually bring home 3 or 4 trophies.

Copyright © 2025 Darryl Vidal

This was a time when these trophies, although not made of precious metal, did feature marble bases, and metal parts, which made them decently heavy. They were much nicer than the plastic on plastic trophies that became more popular, and cheaper to make in the 90s.

Joe started organizing regular trips to tournaments for his students. Every Sunday morning, a caravan of parents and students would gather at Sensei Rosas' house. From there, we would head out together to compete in various events across LA and OC. These trips became a routine part of our lives, fostering a strong sense of camaraderie and shared purpose among the dojo members.

In kata, I began experimenting with creating my own forms that showcased my strengths and preferences. My kata featured high, dramatic kicks and explosive jumping and spinning techniques, which set them apart from the traditional forms.

While most students stuck to the standard school katas, which focused on fundamental movements and lacked the flair, my custom forms stood out for their dynamic and visually striking elements. This distinctive approach made my kata nearly unbeatable in the color belt divisions, where my creativity and technical skill gave me an edge over my competitors.

At one point, I would open the kata by running up to the judges and doing a russian split, double kick high above the heads of the judges seated at the front of the ring. Accompany that with a hearty "KIAI" and that would scare the pants off of most people. Then several spinning and jumping kicks with the loud kiais to keep their attention.

In kumite, my dojo buddies and I developed a reputation for dominating the sparring ring with practical and difficult-to-defend techniques; in some cases, sneaking moves that took full advantage of the rules. We became known for our use of the groin kick, a powerful and effective move that could catch opponents off guard.

Another technique we developed and labeled the "choo choo train" involved closing in on the opponent and unleashing a rapid series of straight punches in a relentless assault. This tactic was designed to overwhelm our opponents and force them out of the ring, and it proved to be a formidable strategy in karate sparring.

I also made effective use of quick, strategic techniques during kumite. A sharp groin shot followed by a precise back-knuckle strike to the face often led to swift victories. These fast, decisive moves allowed me to score points quickly, often winning matches in rapid 1-2-3 sequences. This approach not only secured me frequent victories but also earned me multiple trophies at each tournament.

Overall, my success in both kata and kumite was a reflection of my confidence and creativity. Unsatisfied to compete with the same as everyone else, a little improvisation, sprinkled with some showing off was a recipe for success.

Breaking

As a young karate student, the allure of breaking boards was irresistible. Our backyard became a testing ground, a makeshift dojo where we experimented with various objects. We scavenged for suitable targets, our eyes drawn to the discarded scrap piles of construction sites that dotted our neighborhood. Thin pieces of wood, remnants of forgotten projects, became our primary focus. We discovered that these slender boards, when struck with precision, would shatter with a satisfying crack.

However, as we delved deeper into this newfound distraction, we realized that breaking wasn't merely about brute force. The orientation of the wood played a crucial role. Striking a board along its grain proved to be far easier than breaking it against the grain. Actually, it's almost impossible to break any 12" wide board, thicker than an inch, across the grain. Try it before you tell me you've done it.

We began cutting 12"x 8" x 1" boards; the ideal dimensions for adult breaking boards that won't break without enough snap—combination of speed and power, using kicks, shuto (knife-hand chop), and of course punches. You will learn very quickly that the skin covering your bare knuckles is thin and filled with nerves and blood vessels. Meaning striking with straight punches into hardwood hurts and bleeds a lot—especially if the boards don't break.

As our skills progressed, so did the complexity of our challenges. Board breaking, once a simple act of speed and power, evolved into a meticulous study. We learned to channel our energy, focusing it with laser-like precision. A single misstep, a moment of hesitation, could result in a

Copyright © 2025 Darryl Vidal

failed break and a sting of disappointment—often accompanied by bruised and bloodied knuckles, scratches down the hand and wrist.

Invariably, that means one of these things happened:

1. The holder lost his grip. So now your knuckles are hurt or skinned, and so are his hands, and the boards are still intact. So you must try again, or lose face in front of the crowd and/or lose faith in yourself. Neither are acceptable. But at least you can share blame with the holder.

2. The holder wasn't stable enough, so your speed and power is absorbed by the weak holder. This can mean that the holder must reinforce his stance and arm positions, and/or get help. This means your knuckles are hurt or bleeding, and the boards still are intact. So you must try again, but at least you can blame the holder again.

3. The boards break! Which means you throw your arms up is success, bow to your holders and the crowd, and walk off stage to nurse your wounds.

Copyright © 2025 Darryl Vidal

When the boards break as planned, you come away reeling from adrenaline and bursting with confidence. Now learn to channel and recall that energy.

In all these cases, your knuckles are skinned and bleeding, but a quick visit to the bathroom and a paper towel does the trick to hide your injuries. No need to attract attention, and no want for sympathy.

This is the first level of mind-over-matter development.

Anyone worth their salt watching kung-fu movies and watching Bruce Lee, knows you have to toughen your hands and knuckles. Board breaking is just one of the reasons.

All athlete's bodies adjust and evolve to the rigors of their sport. Baseball players and golfers develop calluses in their palms and the base of their fingers. Martial artists do this with their knuckles. A concept foreign to non-martial artists. Muay Thai fighters and boxers wrap their hands to stabilize their wrists and protect their skin.

So it's mostly traditional karate types who you might see striking a makiwara with bare-knuckles or even punching into sandpaper tacked on the wall.

From there we graduated to breaking multiple boards, learning that two boards are more than double the difficulty of breaking single boards. Three boards being much, much, more difficult, nearly impossible for anyone but an experienced karate master.

This is where energy focus comes into play. The breaker must focus his energy beyond the target—penetration is the key. This is also the most common failure when novices break. Their focus on the target causes them to "short-stroke," meaning they aren't penetrating through the target. I always teach my students to focus on a spot 4 - 6 inches behind the board. This type of visualization enables penetrating power.

In order to break multiple boards with a hand strike or a kick, it requires exacting focus and the mental ability to "know" you can make the break. Any wavering of thought and the failure is not only embarrassing, but extremely painful. If you follow through to try again, you have to ignore the pain and worry of actually breaking bones—this is not for the faint of heart.

The mental aspect of board breaking became as crucial as the physical. We had to cultivate a state of unwavering focus, blocking out distractions and fears. The pain of a missed break, the sting of splintered wood against our skin, became a test of our resolve. It was a lesson in perseverance, teaching us to rise above discomfort and push our limits.

This is the second level of mind-over-matter. Multiple boards require the same precision and focus we mastered with the single board, but now you must amplify the speed and power component. More than double. That means you have to try to triple your power keeping the precision. Can you do it? Have you done it? Keep talking.

Often, we would engage in breaking demonstrations, oblivious to the toll it took on our bodies. Only later, when the adrenaline subsided, would we notice the blood trickling from our wounds. A concerned teammate or family member might point out the injury, their voice tinged with surprise. "Did you know you're bleeding?" they would ask, their question a stark reminder of the physicality of our pursuit.

Spinning, Jumping and Speed Breaks

We started doing demonstrations including breaking at the start of each new karate session, basically every 8 weeks. This gave ample opportunity to experiment with new and different breaking techniques.

The first challenges after the basic chop (shuto aka knife hand) and punching techniques, and adding additional boards of course, included kicks.

I'd often come away from breaking boards with kicks limping with swollen toes or heels.

The reverse shuto (chop starting in front of the body and striking horizontally with the palm-down), as opposed to the shuto or palm-up chop, is not as strong as it is fast. The strike has to be nominal for both speed and power. A fast strike without enough momentum (power) behind it will come to an abrupt stop with a solid board.

Watch for hitting your wrist against the edge of the board. The skin around the wrist is soft and will bleed when scratched or cut.

If you catch the base of the wrist bones (carpal bones) instead of the flesh and muscle around the metacarpals, you can easily displace (dislocate), or break (fracture) one of these bones.

It's always easier to break boards on static mounts, typical cinder blocks. These don't give, although they might cause the boards to bounce and not break.

Part of the difficulty of breaking with kicks is the first and most obvious challenge of accuracy. Kicking someone in the groin or stomach requires just generalized kick placement. Most people can kick someone at these targets without much problem. However, the challenge comes with not only focusing on a smaller target, but with striking with the right part of the foot with enough speed.

Since the leg is such a powerful limb, more often the strike is lumbering, able to knock the wind out of an opponent but not fast enough to snap the board. A poorly placed kick might just push on the holder's arms, so more people are required to hold the boards still and firm. Also, a kick that just uses the sole of the foot doesn't make breaks, for a front kick, you must have extended the ball of the foot forward and the toes back and out of the way. Hitting with

Copyright © 2025 Darryl Vidal

the toes on a front kick can lead to a debilitating and painful broken toe.

If using a sidekick aka knife-edge kick, once again, if the foot isn't angled correctly, the soft heel won't snap the board, and if the toes make any contact, they will break. Round kicks aren't conducive to breaking because like the knuckles, the skin atop the instep of the foot is soft and will bruise easily.

It also becomes more important that the person, or persons holding the board get their fingers out of the way because the errant kick will invariably hit their fingers, which can be quite painful for the holder. The new challenge for the board holder becomes extending their arms fully, for maximum strength, and folding their fingers away from the center of the boards. Typically a second person is added either to back up the primary holder, or to get a second pair of hands on the boards, creating four posts for added strength and stability, and twice as many fingers to smash on accident.

Next in the progression of difficulty was the spinning technique. Spinning with a reverse shuto (knife-hand chop) was pretty easy and yet impressive. It takes a modicum of balance and footwork to do the reverse spin (around the blind-side) and land the reverse chop in a horizontal strike.

The back-hook kick becomes the next, more daunting challenge. This is the blind-side spinning kick that Bruce Lee does a hundred times in Enter the Dragon. By spinning through the blind-side, the leg is chambered and sweeps across the target. For karate sparring, it works to hit your opponent with the sole of the foot, but for breaking, the sole of the foot is too soft. You must strike with either the bottom of the heel, or the back of the heel. I will tell you, both of those parts of the foot will bruise after breaking boards, and if the boards don't break, you'll be limping off that foot for at least several days.

Some karate people never develop a decent enough back-hook kick to pull off this break. My back-hook kicks were smooth as silk. I could hit with the toes, sole, or heel as I wished. I used to joke that I could pull your eyelashes with my toes doing a back-hook kick. So of course, the next evolution for breaking would be the jumping back-hook. As lithe as I was in my teens and twenties, I could jump back-spin and break two boards on targets over six-feet high. This demo was very impressive when I would have a holder stand atop a chair and hold the board a foot over my head. I still have old videos of doing this break.

I soon took my breaking demonstrations to another level by incorporating speed breaks, which required a different level of precision and power. Unlike traditional breaking techniques where the materials are supported, speed breaks rely entirely on the momentum of the strike to break the object which has no inertia. I started holding boards with one hand and punching through them with the other, showing control and force in a single motion. This is the way O'Hara breaks the board in Enter the Dragon. When Bruce Lee comments, "Boards don't hit back!"

One of my favorite techniques involved setting a brick vertically on a stack of bricks and using a sideways shuto (chop) strike to snap it in half. These speed breaks were particularly impressive because they showcased the power generated by pure technique, without the aid of support, further pushing the boundaries of what I could do in my demonstrations. It is common to cut or scrape my hands during these demonstrations so oftentimes I would finish with cut wrists and bloody knuckles.

The other popular speed break was to line up up to four vertical cement blocks and speed break them with a side kick. This one will leave you with a sore or swollen heel in all instances.

I began incorporating board and brick breaking demonstrations into my martial arts demonstration repertoire as a way to showcase the power and precision I had developed through years of training. These demonstrations became an exciting part of my participation at karate tournaments. Since I had gotten to know many of the tournament promoters personally, I would approach them during events and ask if I could perform a brief demo in the downtime between kata competitions and kumite. There was usually a short delay in the proceedings anyway, and my demo became a way to keep the audience entertained while adding some excitement to the event.

For these demos, I would bring along boards, bricks, and even a rock for the finale. The breaking demonstrations were thrilling for the audience, who watched in anticipation as I lined up my materials. I would start by breaking several boards, usually stacked on top of one another, with a well-placed strike or kick. The audience always responded with gasps and applause, especially when the boards split cleanly in two. I would then move on to bricks, which were more challenging but even more impressive when they crumbled under a precise blow.

Rock Breaking

It was in my backyard in Chino where I first experimented with breaking rocks. The first obstacle one must navigate before attempting the rock break is mental. It's that mind-over-matter thing again.

If you look at a rock, and hold it in your hand, you can feel the density and the inherent hardness of the rock. In your logical mind, you can't believe it could be broken by hand. Nothing in the practical, everyday world would lead you to believe that a person could break a rock with just his hand. But if you don't believe it can be done, then you better not try it. The consequences could be painful and even debilitating. Mas Oyama's book "This is Karate" shows not how to do it, but just shows a bunch of rocks that he and his student break. Some of them are unbelievable. But that's the point.

By this time, I was preparing for my Sho Dan test and quite confident in myself. I'd already been breaking boards and cement blocks for years and experimenting with different styles of breaks. I believed if I could speed-break a cement block, then I must be able to break a rock. And if Oyama could do it, maybe I could. Although I wouldn't be getting into the ring with a bull anytime soon.

The rocks shown in the Oyama books were massive, but that didn't stop me, it made me look harder at what I could try first. I made a point to drive around town to see where I could find rocks. It tended to be riverbeds, and of course, the beach!

The riverbed near my house in Chino was a wash that was normally dry unless it was actively raining. All sorts of rock littered the wash and made for a grand variety for me to explore. Unfortunately, every rock looked impossible to break. What was I thinking?

Weather rounded or flat, rough or smooth, they just seemed totally unbreakable. I started by looking for oblong rocks with at least one flat side that I would hit with my hand. Once I found one, I would throw it down on another bigger rock to see if they would break. Surprisingly, an oblong rock, not too thick, when thrown correctly to hit another rock at its halfway point would shatter. The question was, can you hit it that hard?.

Copyright © 2025 Darryl Vidal

I later learned that not all rocks are the same when it comes to breaking them. Igneous rocks, like granite for instance, are very hard and have no layers, which is denser and doesn't just crack down the middle. Sedimentary rocks are made of compressed sand and will crumble - not making for an impressive demo. Granite rocks are so hard that they would often shatter upon impact, splintering unpredictably, instead of breaking in two nice pieces. In contrast, limestone rocks could be sizable, and breakable. Limestone rocks would break clean, making them more suitable for controlled demonstrations. So it really came down to where I was looking.

Because of this I would specifically avoid granite rocks, and sites where they seemed to be the most common.

One time, while preparing for a breaking demo, I went to a location where I could only find granite rocks in the hilly riverbeds descending from the hills in Alta Loma. Since they would need to be smaller and thinner, they weren't as impressive to look at, but I knew they would be much harder to break. Finally, I gathered two or three rocks that looked breakable, even though they were granite. They were oblong and flat, so I thought they might work.

Unfortunately, the inability to find a nice limestone metamorphic rock planted a seed of doubt in my mind.

When it was demo time, I went through the normal progression of doing some board breaks, punches, chops and kicks. A spin kick into a jump kick. Then the brick breaks. Usually all speed breaks. Then, time for the finale.

The highlight of the demo was always the rock break. I practiced the technique relentlessly until I could confidently break a rock with a single strike. For the audience, this was the ultimate demonstration of what martial arts training could achieve—turning the body into a powerful weapon capable of breaking through even the hardest materials. But there's always the Bruce Lee quote, "Boards don't hit back!" And neither do rocks!

I usually stopped the demo and did a little background speech about how hard it is to break a rock. That it is a true practice of mind over matter. I prepared the break by stacking up the bricks that I had previously broken into a pile about thigh high. I placed the rock on top of the pile.

I always made a point out of doing a meditation and focus routine consisting of kneeling and meditating. I would literally focus my mind on the rock and hold it and rotate it in my hands looking for the perfect grip. The mental technique I use is to hit the rock as if my hand was a hammer, which means I have to hit the rock with my right hand chop while holding it with my left hand, as hard as I could, even if it would break my hand.

I would do several ritualistic practice strikes, raising my hand, and mimicking the slow-motion chop. After several anticipation building practice strikes, I raised my hand and smashed the rock with a full kiai. Tiny specks of rock shattered off, but the rock remained in one large piece. Adrenaline pumping, I took another deep breath, fixed my grip on the rock and went at it again with full force and even more intensity.

Once again, shards of the rock scattered, but it remained more or less whole.

The audience held their collective breath waiting to see what happened next. Finally, on my third strike, I mustered all my energy and mental focus and smashed the rock as hard as I could.

The granite rock shattered into a million pieces, with shards and fragments flying all over the gym floor. The crowd clapped, and I stood up in a daze, my energy and focus making my head spin. They had to call the janitor to sweep up the shards of broken rock scattered across the floor, but I just walked off the stage in a daze coming down from the adrenaline rush.

Then the promoter came to shake my hand and noticed that there was a trail of blood following me. On that third strike, the rock had mistakenly rested atop my pinky finger. The final blow smashed the inner side of my pinky, and I could see a wide gash and a white chalky material beyond the split flesh. More work for the janitor.

It wasn't quite gushing, but I had to run to the bathroom to find enough paper towels to keep from making a much larger mess.

I wrapped it with tape and went home without competing in the kumite competition. My mother, who was a medical assistant, recommended I take a trip to the emergency room.

You know how it is at the ER, waiting behind all the sick people, old people in gurneys and crying babies. After several hours waiting, the doctor cut off the tape I had wrapped around my finger and said, "Hmmm."

He took out a syringe and injected pain-killers directly into the split in my finger, about four-or-five times up and down the gash. My finger was already numb but it was still quite a site to look at. I ended up needing five stitches to close it up. You can still see the faint scar inside my left pinky today. But I did break the rock into a million pieces.

Once I went to the beach and on my way to leave I went to find some "breakers." Most of the rocks were smaller so I ended up bringing home about five smaller smooth rounded limestone rocks. Although small, they were perfect breakers because of their shape which allowed me a nice grip with my left hand and a smooth top for me to hit.

So for the next demo, I only had these smaller rocks, so I took four of them and broke them in quick succession, one after the other. It became so easy, I began doing breaking demos where I would explain that I would break the rock without hitting it hard. I would tell the audience that I may have to hit the rock two or three times, if it didn't break the first time, I would start hitting it harder. These demos weren't very good. If you have to explain why you're doing something, the audience loses interest. That's true for any type of demonstration. So the bigger the rock, the better.

It became a side hobby of mine. Anytime I went to the beach, before leaving I would gather a select few narrow and oblong rocks that would be candidates to be broken, and scatter them in my front porch garden. Even today, there is a collection of oblong flat rocks that decorate my porch for that time that I would need them for a breaking demonstration—and every time I look at them I know I can break them!

Early Hobbies

Skateboarding was a passion that I shared with my brother, Irwin. We spent countless hours practicing tricks and exploring the city streets. Our early attempts at building our own skateboards from plywood were ambitious but ultimately unsuccessful. We soon realized that saving up for the necessary parts was a more practical approach.

As we got better, we ventured to the iconic skateparks of the Inland Empire, such as Willow Skatepark and Upland Pipeline. While we mastered the basics of street freestyle skating, the vertical pools and half-pipes remained a challenge for us. Nevertheless, the thrill of gliding through the skatepark and conquering new tricks was an unforgettable experience.

We built our own skateboard ramps on the side of our house that had a long runway. All the local kids would come over and hit the ramp.

Shooting Sports

My father was a strong supporter of our hobbies, and he encouraged our interest in archery and shooting. With limited space, our backyard became our shooting range. We would set up cardboard boxes against the fence for archery practice and target shooting with our pellet rifles. Our creativity knew no bounds as we improvised with various objects for targets, aiming at anything that caught our fancy at the nearby farm.

While our parents were away, we indulged in a more adventurous pastime: shooting at birds perched on trees and fences. It was a thrilling but risky activity that we engaged in with a sense of youthful rebellion.

Despite the occasional mishap or parental scolding, our archery and shooting adventures were filled with joy and excitement. We learned valuable skills and developed a sense of practice for improvement. The little backyard range was our playground, where we experimented and pushed our boundaries. I became so accurate with my .177 pellet rifle, I could hit worms and bugs at 30 feet (our backyard wasn't that big). We'd live to shoot targets that exploded. Shooting at paper was boring. We even experimented with moving targets—swinging targets on a string and timing the shot.

As an adult I am an active shooter of both pistols and rifles. I believe as a martial artist guns are the ultimate martial weapon and we must either master them, or fear them.

Electronics

As I started writing this book, there are events in my life I haven't even recalled until now—and wouldn't imagine I'd write about. They're mostly innocuous; inconsequential. But it does reveal a nuance of my eclectic identity. Likely because my father knew I was mechanically, or logically inclined, he also fostered this aptitude with electronics.

Funny thing about the 1970s and 80s is there wasn't much around in terms of electronic toys or consumer oriented electronics. The most advanced personal electronics of the era would be a transistor radio.

On a trip to the local Radio Shack (Google it if you don't know this franchise), I saw a little electronics kit made by Heathkit to make an AM radio (Google it if you don't know this is). They actually offered several kits which I ended up making including light sequencers and amplifiers for the radio.

Connections were made on a breadboard (perforated circuit board) and solder. Which means you need to be able to read schematics, identify components, and learn to use a soldering iron—which is an art of its own.

My most significant accomplishment with these was when my father decided we would build our own Personal Computer (1982ish). This was a massive project. The entirety of a PC-DOS machine with 64Kb of RAM and 5.25" floppy drives.

After twenty or so separate schematics and soldering thousands of transistors, resistors, capacitors, and a Cathode Ray Tube that could kill you if you touch it wrong, I did it.

I could now run an early version of DOS and play simple games, and I had a word processor and spreadsheet.

This was all text-based—no graphics. I learned a ton, and developed some skills that gave me awesome technical information and insight into electronics fabrication and personal computer operations.

Little did we envision that all these thousands of components would just be printed using gold on a non-conducting substrate—like printing stamps. Basically today, that PC, but with over 10,000 times the computing power, is stamped onto a piece of fiberglass and sold for about $200.

Fishing

From an early age, I developed a love for fishing. Though my actual experiences were limited to family camping trips and occasional outings on a boat with my uncle, there was something about fishing that captivated me. It felt like an instinctive draw, an unexplainable pull that kept me wanting more, even when my opportunities were few and far between.

When I was in grade school, I heard rumors about a pond that was within bicycle riding distance from my house. Intrigued, I started visiting the pond on my own. It took a few trips to get things right—finding the right kind of pole, learning about the best bait, and figuring out how to use a bobber—but once I had my setup down, I was hooked. I would gather worms, pack my gear, and head to the pond, where I could catch Bluegill in abundance. I'd ride home proudly with my catch, and my mother would fry them up for dinner. Those early fishing trips became more than just a pastime; they were moments of independence and discovery, nurturing my connection to nature and the simple pleasures of life.

When we moved to Chino, my passion for fishing remained strong. I would study maps meticulously, searching for the nearest lakes and daydreaming about the chance to spend time on the water, casting lines and catching fish. I hoped that our family would make frequent trips to these lakes, but my father had a different idea in mind. He enjoyed boating more than fishing, which led us down a different path.

His first purchase was a small sailboat—a dinghy—that we would wrestle onto the roof of our car and haul to the nearest lake. He also bought a little paperback book of how to sail. Between this book and being on the water in Lake Puddingstone, I learned how to sail during those trips, navigating the little boat across the water, but I still couldn't shake the desire to fish. Then, my father upgraded to a jet boat, and we all learned how to water ski, speeding across lakes and rivers. While these trips were filled with excitement, they didn't allow me to indulge in the peaceful, solitary pursuit of fishing that I craved. Despite being on the water, fishing remained out of reach as my father's love for boating took center stage.

Once I started working at Hughes Aircraft Company alongside my father and brother, I was introduced to my brother's friend, Scott, a passionate fisherman. Scott's enthusiasm for the sport was infectious, and I eagerly joined him on his camping and fishing trips to the Sierra Nevada mountains. Scott was the consummate camp host that would wholeheartedly invite anyone along and loan them anything they needed. He just charged a donation for the campsite and supplies and invited anyone to bring along their own gear and guns.

Our adventures along the Kern River and Bishop Creeks were filled with the thrill of casting my line and the anticipation of a catch. I quickly learned the art of trout fishing, mastering the use of ultralight tackle and Panther Martin spinners. These small, brightly colored lures proved to be incredibly effective, allowing me to catch and release countless trout without harming them.

Something that I am most affected by is creeks and rivers. Although I love a great mountain lake, I'll take a stream to wade and fish anytime. But alas, if I was really dedicated to fishing, I'd have a boat, but there's so many reasons I never bought a boat that it's not really worth writing about. It would just be me listing lame excuse after lame excuse.

One of my first trips to the Sierras coincided with my birthday in May. From that year on, I made it a tradition to embark on a Sierra fishing trip on my special day. These annual retreats became my "Coming to Jesus" times, as the serene beauty of the mountains and the tranquility of the creeks provided a spiritual connection to nature. During these trips, I would often engage in meaningful conversations with my children, discussing their beliefs and exploring the concept of God.

Over the years, I've expanded my fishing pursuits to include bass fishing with plastics, crankbaits and, most notably, fly fishing—considered the pinnacle of artificial lure fishing. The delicate art of casting a fly, mimicking the natural movements of aquatic insects, has become a deeply satisfying and rewarding aspect of my fishing exploits.

My oldest son and I recently explored Upper Kern river; the Northern section of the wild Southern Sierra river that drains into Lake Isabella. It was initially one of the first rivers I fished with Scott. But after years fishing both the Kern and Bishop Creeks, I began to focus more on the Bishop Creeks area and less making the shorter trip to Kern.

This trip was a re-enactment of one of the first camping and fishing trips I had taken with just him and I, when he was 4 or 5. It took a while to find the right spot but in the end we limited-out for two days. The difference was we were 30 years older, and we were both re-discovering the track after that span.

As it turned out, the river was stocked the morning we arrived. Lesson: Always check the fish planting schedule.

Skiing

Growing up in Southern California, skiing was a foreign concept to our family. It seemed like a sport reserved for the wealthy; a luxury beyond our reach. However, my brother Irwin's decision to join the ski club at school piqued my interest. I wanted to be cool like him, so I decided to give it a try.

With ski resorts like Mount Baldy, Wrightwood, and Big Bear within driving distance, we had ample opportunity to explore this exclusive winter sport. After Irwin's first few trips, we started going on our own, eventually investing in our own gear. As experienced skateboarders, we discovered that our natural balance and skill on the board translated surprisingly well to the slopes.

While Irwin was always better and faster than me, I did my best to keep up. Skiing became a shared passion that brought us closer together.

After Irwin left for the Army, I continued to pursue skiing with my friends in college. I developed my skills to the point where I was able to ski parallel and even tackle the black diamond slopes (the black diamond slopes in Southern California are nothing like black diamond slopes elsewhere).

Skiing became more than just a sport for me; it was a way to challenge myself, connect with nature, and enjoy the thrill of adventure. Although I never did ski outside of Southern California until much later.

Snowboarding

After having our first children, skiing became a bit of a luxury. So it wasn't' until Justin was 7 and Bradley was 5 that I decided we'd start snowboarding. Our first time up renting gear was always a little challenging, but we quickly acquired the gear for the boys and within that first year, we were going to the local ski resort almost every Saturday. With my skateboarding experience I led the way up and down the hills. The boys learned quickly and it became our favorite winter activity.

As the girls got to age, I brought them up and by the time Nissa-Belle was 5, all the kids were grooming up the slopes, and the boys were doing their best tricking. It was about this time I'd started planning annual trips to Mammoth Mountain in the Eastern Sierras and it was always a hit.

We had our share of incidents and minor accidents either on the slope or off, but it wasn't until the boys were in their teens that we started to accumulate more significant injuries.

I prided myself with rarely falling, because I didn't try difficult terrain or tricks. I could handle the SoCal black diamonds but I never did jumps or rails. It only took one fall from the beginner's half-pipe at Mammoth to learn I was too old to learn to make the drastic turn required at each side of the pipe, so I was a groomer from that point on. I can say that we all went down Cornice, a famous vertical run at Mammoth. But that was a one-time deal.

About the same time, the boys, getting more and more confident, began to rack up the broken bones. Brad broke his collarbone one year, then the other the following year. I had at least a couple of broken ribs and a dislocated collar-bone. Justin, after taking a break to start having kids, blew his knee out jumping.

Once COVID hit, everything changed. Condo rates doubled and lift ticket prices went even higher. Years before, I could pay for the trip and a couple of days for everyone on the slopes. After, I started telling everyone, they have to pay for their own tickets. Then there was the one year.

It wasn't our first blizzard, a couple of years previous, a storm came through and they warned us to prepare to be snowed in for 3-4 days. So shortly after setting up, we left.

The spinout must have been 2017 or 2018 when another atmospheric river hit the Sierras. It was white-out conditions as we headed home in two separate cars. Myself and April in my BMW X6, and Shain, her husband Jon, Brad and his girlfriend in April's Ford Edge.

We were slowly making our way South on 395 just North of Independence at around 20 mph full blizzard conditions. I led the way, when I decided to try to pass a slower driver in front. As I crossed the divider, which was also its own little snow bank, the rear wheels spun and so did we. A couple of spins on the highway and we ended up facing the wrong way on 395. Jon and the kids behind, watched in awe as I spun, stopped, turned around, and continued South down the highway as if nothing had happened. Of course, April was in a state of shock. So bad that we haven't ventured back for our Winter getaway to Mammoth since.

Brad and the girls continue to love to snowboard. In 2024, recovering from a hip replacement was the first year I missed snowboarding completely for 30 years. I don't want to be done with the sport but my body may not agree. We'll have to see what Winter 2025-26 brings.

Golf

Through the first half (so far) of my life, golf would be a mostly foreign, even innocuous sport to me. I never held a golf club, or stepped on a golf course. It just wasn't a thing until I started working in the corporate world. After being in the workforce for several years working with professional sales people and corporate entities, I could see that a lot of "business" was actually done on the golf course.

I had been invited to play, but never accepted because—obviously—I would make a fool out of myself. Thus I decided that when I turned 30 I would learn to play golf.

For my 30th birthday my wife would buy me my first set of clubs and I would begin the arduous journey along with many other golfers, seeking the ability to hit a tiny ball with a long metal club thousands of yards. It always amazed me that my skills as a martial artist lend nothing, toward swinging a golf club.

I engaged my Apple buddy, Glenn, to help me get started playing golf. We've been golf buddies for 30 years now.

Life Changing Event

Although I never considered it at the time, my early 20's was marred by a life-changing event. By early 1986, my competitive karate career was waning. I was coming out of a splash of fame from the karate kid and was considered more of a celebrity than a competitor. In addition, the competition got wise to my methods and everyone and their brother started incorporating more acrobatics, jumping, flying and spinning moves into their katas. New categories of kata called Showmanship or Musical kata were added and the competition became—competitive. My visits to the local tournaments were more about signing autographs and greeting fans rather than competing with them.

The event would happen at a tournament hosted by my sensei Joe Rosas at the Chino High School Gym.

Working to promote the event as a world-class open karate tournament, Joe engaged with several of the top promoters and arbitrators of the time. Joe recruited Ron Chapel as tournament Director, and Frank Trejo and Billy Blanks to appear and do a demonstration. This was before Billy's breakthrough Tae-Bo.

Being part of the tournament operations I wasn't planning on competing. I was there more for appearances sake but since I was there, Joe encouraged me to join the kata and sparring competitions so the audience could see "the guy who was in the Karate Kid movie" do the kata that made him famous.

As I stretched and prepared for the kata, I just did a light run through of the kata. I always hate stretching and after years of competing, I started a bad habit of not stretching until the last few minutes before competing. I thought to myself, "go in cold and hit it hard."

The first move in my kata was intended to wake up the judges from their semi-boredom from watching and scoring kata competitors for hours. I would start at the center of the ring and make the requisite announcements, then I would run up and do a Russian-split jumping double front kick just over the heads of the seated judges. It was a sure fire way of getting their attention and led to many kata wins.

This time however, going in without stretching took its toll. I ran up and planted my feet for the vertical jump into the Russian-splits jump and my left knee blew out. I heard a loud, sickening snap and fell to the ground.

I had never had a knee problem in the past and didn't know what happened. Only it felt like my knee exploded. I regained my balance and went through the rest of the kata without doing any of the jump kicks—of which there were at least four. As I hobbled through the rest of the kata my knee collapsed at least 2 more times.

Although obviously in pain and injured, I played it off as best as I could and pretended everything was fine. I can't even recall if I placed in the competition.

Back sitting on the stands, my fiance-at-the-time came over concerned. She knew I was injured and encouraged me to pack up and go to the emergency room. But since I was able to get back and walk around, I stubbornly decided not to go.

The next day my knee looked like a football—swollen and purple. So I went to the doctor. He did the usual ACL and PCL pulling test and said that I had likely torn both. He put me in a full-length cast. I was getting married in four weeks.

Although I was to wear it for six weeks, my wedding was scheduled for July 19th, so two-weeks early, I went in and told them to cut it off so I could walk down the aisle.

I wasn't that stable, but I did walk down the aisle. In fact, on our honeymoon in Mazatlan, I actually paraglided and landed safely on the beach with my lame knee and all.

Weeks later I would go in for an arthroscopy. The doctor would clean up the torn meniscus but leave the torn ligaments as they were, ACL— detached, PCL mostly torn. The alternatives at the time were cadaver ligaments or goretex. Neither option seemed advisable. When the doctor is iffy, go with the instinct. He said with this injury, I can go on without the ligament with some good physical therapy. The alternative would be reconstruction, several major incisions, and questionable results.

The doctor convinced me that I could mostly recover my movement with therapy and would have minimal additional problems without having a major knee reconstruction.

I did not know at the time how my life would be affected by the injury, but 40 years later, my right hip would be plagued by osteoarthritis and need a hip arthroplasty.

Ego, Alter Ego

The Emergence of Ego

As a teenager, I was on the cusp of discovering who I was, and like many adolescents, I found myself caught in the intricate dance between confidence and doubt. My ego was bolstered by a series of small triumphs that seemed to affirm my place in the world. I was an A student, effortlessly gliding through my classes with minimal effort, a fact that did not go unnoticed by my peers or teachers. I wasn't just smart; I was academically gifted. This innate ability to excel in school became one of the cornerstones of my self-esteem. It felt like a natural part of me, something that I could rely on without question.

Outside of the classroom, I trained in karate and wrestling, two disciplines that further reinforced my sense of self. Karate, with its emphasis on focus and physical prowess, gave me a structured way to channel my energy and hone my skills. Wrestling, with its demand for both mental and physical endurance, added another layer to my growing sense of capability. These activities, combined with my academic success, inflated my ego. I started to see myself as someone who could succeed in any arena I entered (except tall-people sports). I was confident, perhaps even a little cocky, and I wore this confidence like armor.

Despite my expanding ego, I never fully aligned myself with the sports and athletics crowd. I wasn't the type to hang out exclusively with jocks, although I had friends within that group. But as an immigrant family, we didn't inherently follow mainstream American sports like Baseball, Football and Basketball. I did play these sports in the streets and fields but I didn't grow up following the normal teams from San Diego, the Padres, Chargers and temporarily, the Clippers. This missing link always kept me from being a true "sports fan." Which probably didn't really affect my social life, although the lack of having a "My Team" still leaves me out of many sports discussions when caught up in general social situations.

Despite this fact, I made friends easily across all cliques. My versatility in navigating different social circles became another point of pride. I could be friendly with the athletes, chat with the brainiacs, and still find common ground with the artsy crowd. Yet, there was always a part of me that remained slightly detached, never fully committing to any one group. I was confident in who I was, but at the same time, I was a bit of an outsider—comfortable, but not entirely at home in any one place.

The Teenage Facade

While I projected confidence, some might call conceit, there was one area where I felt decidedly less sure of myself—around girls. It wasn't that I was completely awkward or shy; I could engage in conversation and be charming when I needed to be. But there was an underlying discomfort that I couldn't quite shake. It wasn't until I was a senior in high school that I began to feel more at ease in the presence of the opposite sex. Even then, it was more of an act than genuine confidence. I learned how to play the part, to say the right things, to appear self-assured, but inside, I was still that unsure kid, second-guessing myself at every turn.

The ability to mask my insecurities became a skill in itself. I realized that I could project an image of someone who was completely in control, even when I wasn't. This act became a part of my everyday life, a performance that I refined over time. But behind the bravado, there was a constant sense of unease, a feeling that I was merely pretending to be something I was not. This duality between the confident exterior and the uncertain interior marked the beginning of a lifelong struggle—a battle between ego and alter ego.

The Birth of the Alter Ego

Even as my ego swelled with each success, there was another part of me that quietly whispered doubts. This was my alter ego, the voice of my insecurities, the part of me that felt like an imposter in my own life. Long before I ever heard the term "imposter syndrome," I was living it. Despite my achievements, I often felt like I didn't truly belong, like I was faking it and that one day, someone would figure it out.

In karate, for example, I was good, but I knew that there were others who were better. My training took place at a Parks and Recreation department, not at a prestigious karate studio. Our style was an offshoot of Chinese Kenpo, a style that was difficult to define in both style and lineage. It didn't carry the weight or recognition of other, more established martial arts. This nagged at me, making me feel like my accomplishments in karate were somehow less valid. I wasn't training with the elite karate schools, so how could I consider myself truly skilled? My alter ego fed on these doubts, growing stronger with each passing year. What I didn't recognize at the time was I was training with the best. Although never one to proclaim one martial art superior over another, there are aspects of our own Chinese, or more accurately, Hawaiian Kenpo, than other forms of better known styles of Kenpo. I will not delve deeper into this in this book as it would be politically volatile to tackle this subject in the public square.

The Academic Divide

This feeling of being an imposter extended to other areas of my life as well. While I excelled in school, I was acutely aware that I wasn't the smartest kid in the room. I was good, yes, but there were always others who seemed to grasp concepts more quickly, who could solve problems faster, and who didn't need to work as hard to maintain their grades. These individuals were few and far between, but it seemed that each of my classes included one of these "even smarter" kids. These kids all went directly to universities, some even to Ivy League—this was an utter embarrassment.

I knew how to play the academic game, how to study efficiently and get good grades, but deep down, I felt like I was just keeping up rather than truly excelling. I was just jogging alongside the high achievers, not wanting to commit more and risk more.

This sense of inadequacy only deepened as I pursued higher education.

I completed my business bachelor's degree at Cal State University—a respectable institution, but not an Ivy League school. I knew that I was receiving a solid education, but there was always a part of me that wondered if I could have done more, if I could have aimed higher.

The fact that I was attending classes at night while working during the day only added to my sense of being less than. I wasn't fully immersed in the college experience; I was balancing responsibilities, trying to make it all work. My ego reminded me constantly that I was doing well, but my alter ego showed me that it was not as good as I could have, if only my efforts were more directed.

Stepping Into the Workforce

After college, I landed a great job at Hughes Aircraft Company, one of the largest defense contractors of the time. My dad was a maintenance supervisor there working on his second retirement, and he helped me get my foot in the door. Little did I know how key this move was toward my future career in technology.

Copyright © 2025 Darryl Vidal

I started out working with the analog and digital circuits local to the massive Fullerton, California campus, interconnecting 3002 circuits and T-1 lines. Later in those years we started installing a thick orange cable called "ethernet."

This opportunity should have been a confidence boost, and in many ways, it was. I was getting my feet wet in technology systems, learning about telecommunications, and gaining valuable experience in a field that was rapidly evolving.

By 1984, in addition to the other distractions that were occurring in my life, Steve Jobs would introduce the Macintosh computer. In this time, computers and PCs were still not predominant in home life. The most advanced devices at home were digital alarm clocks, televisions, and VCRs. In business it was the digital copier, digital phone systems and facsimile (fax) machines.

Personal Computers were starting to make inroads in business and this is what drove the vast expansion of IBM PCs which overtook the Apple II because of the business focus acceptance of MS-DOS.

I was one of those captivated by the girl with the sledgehammer spinning and smashing the jumbo screen as the Ridley Scott commercial for the Macintosh hit almost every television screen in the US during the 1984 Super Bowl. I had to have one. Not the girl, the computer.

Hughes Aircraft offered an employee loan program to incentivize employees to purchase a personal computer. All our team in Telecommunications opted for the IBM PC. I went for the Mac—I was the only one of my buddies to get one. So the whole thing of sharing pirated software was out the door for me.

But the Mac could do things the PC and MS-DOS couldn't—the Mac was GUI based. DOS was still text-based. The IBM PC fully configured, with printer, was just under $2,000, but the Macintosh, with printer, was $3,200.

I was able to use the Mac effectively for both school and work, even using a Pascal compiler for my programming class.

I was a Mac person for the next several years and once I had started to meet Apple Sales people and Apple System engineers that would call on my company, where I was the IT Analyst, I sought to get a job at the cool, fruit-named company.

I joined during what might be considered the heyday of Apple Computer. Riding the tide of the Macintosh and the Mac SE, I was there to help promote the Mac II (color), System 7, the Apple Newton and the Apple PowerBooks. For a while it was a great place to work.

Only now do I recognize the significance of how this venture affected the course of my life. The System Engineer job I got at Apple was based in San Diego—my favorite town. It would be impossible to commute from Chino, where April and I were living in 1987 in our first home, so we sought to find a new place to raise our growing family.

This is what brought us to the little-known gem in the valley on the route to San Diego known as Highway 395. Later this would become a section of the Interstate 15 Freeway providing a direct route from the Inland Empire to San Diego via Lake Elsinore and Esconidido. The new city was called Murrieta. Where both April and I would start as the first Dance and Karate teachers for the new city.

I thrived in my new role as Sr. System Engineer for Apple Computer and began supporting the Education and Commercial teams as the expert of all things Macintosh. At this time, Apple Computer was the number one employer in the US—It was kind of a big deal. Even to this day, I am involved with the technology systems of the school district I was first introduced to in 1988.

Yet, even in this new role, my alter ego was ever-present. I wasn't a computer science major like my peers on the Apple System Engineering team—I was a business major. While I was learning on the job and performing well, there was always a nagging doubt that I wasn't truly qualified, that I was out of my depth.

My colleagues were experts in their fields, many of them with technical degrees that seemed to place them on a different level. Many of them came from other manufacturers and were polished business people with years of experience.

I was the young guy that came from the aerospace client company. I had no field sales or marketing experience. I knew that I had a lot to offer, but I couldn't shake the feeling that I was somehow faking it, that I didn't really belong in this world of technology and innovation.

It was at Apple where I would refine my business communications and presentation skills which would become the basis of my consultative approach. These skills would be fundamental for operations of a technology consulting firm for the next 20 years of my career after leaving Apple.

The Struggle Within

This internal struggle between my ego and alter ego became a defining feature of my personality. On the one hand, I had accomplished a lot early. I was reasonably successful academically, I was a black belt instructor, I played in a band, I was building a career, I had a growing family, and owned my home.

My ego told me that I was doing well, that I was on the right track, and that I had every reason to be proud of what I had achieved.

But on the other hand, my alter ego continued to sow seeds of doubt. It reminded me that I wasn't the best I could be. I could put in more hours at work and put in a greater effort. But getting home in time to read to the kids was more important than what the sales people wanted.

Alter ego pointed out there were always others who were smarter, more talented, more dedicated, more experienced. It pointed out the shortcomings in my accomplishments—the fact that I trained at a Parks and Recreation department instead of a prestigious karate dojo, the fact that I went to a Cal State instead of an Ivy League school, the fact that I got my job through my father rather than purely on my own merits. This voice of doubt was relentless, and it kept me grounded, perhaps too grounded. It prevented me from fully embracing my successes, from feeling truly confident in my abilities.

Moving Forward

As I continued to navigate the complexities of adulthood, the battle between my ego and alter ego remained unresolved. There were moments when my ego would take the lead, propelling me forward with confidence and determination. But just as often, my alter ego would pull me back, reminding me of my limitations, of the things I still had to learn, of the ways in which I fell short.

This tension between confidence and doubt became a constant in my life. It pushed me to work harder, to strive for excellence, to never settle for mediocrity. But it also held me back, keeping me from fully believing in myself and my abilities. The duality of ego and alter ego is something that I have come to accept as part of who I am. It drives me to achieve, but it also keeps me humble, aware that there is always more to learn, more to do, and more to become.

In the end, the struggle between ego and alter ego is not one that I expect to resolve completely. It is an ongoing journey, one that shapes my decisions, my actions, and my understanding of myself. As I move forward, I do so with the knowledge that both aspects of my identity—my ego and my alter ego—play crucial roles in defining who I am and who I aspire to be.

The Foundation of Cross-Training

The foundation of my martial arts journey was built in high school, where I found myself balancing the rigorous demands of wrestling, karate, Wing Chun, and later, boxing. Each of these disciplines played a crucial role in shaping who I was, both as a martial artist and as a person.

While wrestling provided a strong physical foundation, it was my training in Wing Chun that introduced me to the deeper, more philosophical aspects of martial arts. My introduction to Wing Chun came through a high school buddy who lived and trained with one of Bruce Lee's students. This connection was like striking gold.

Bruce Lee's influence was legendary, and the idea of learning a martial art that he had mastered was exhilarating.

Wing Chun was different from anything I had experienced in wrestling or karate. It was less about brute strength and more about precision, timing, and using an opponent's force against them. The emphasis on close-range combat and efficiency of movement was fascinating to me. My friend and I would spend hours after school practicing "chi sao" together, going over drills, and perfecting our forms. We trained in his garage, which doubled as our makeshift dojo, surrounded by the sounds of Bruce Lee's iconic movies playing in the background.

I actually built a makeshift Wing Chun dummy, called a Mook Jong, out of metal and wood scraps from around the house. Instead of a wooden leg, I used garage door springs. The arms were made from full-round dowels filed down and held in place with rope.

Training in Wing Chun also introduced me to the concept of "chi," the internal energy that martial artists seek to harness and control. It was a new way of thinking about combat and my own physicality. While wrestling had been about exerting maximum effort, Wing Chun was about achieving maximum efficiency with minimal effort.

In karate we called this mastery of internal energy "ki" and it was learned and expressed through the kiai, and breathing methods encompassing the aerobic and anaerobic aspects of mind-over-matter.

This was a profound shift in my approach to martial arts, one that would influence all my future training.

As my skills developed, I earned my brown belt in karate and began teaching regularly as an assistant instructor under Rosas. This was a pivotal transition for me. Teaching required a different set of skills than training or competing. I had to learn how to communicate effectively, break down complex techniques, and be patient with students who were just starting out.

Assisting in the dojo also gave me a new level of responsibility. I wasn't just training for myself anymore; I was helping others on their martial arts journey. This experience deepened my understanding of karate and reinforced the importance of fundamentals. I began to appreciate the balance between physical prowess and mental clarity that karate demanded. As an instructor, I had to embody the principles I was teaching, which meant holding myself to a higher standard both in and out of the dojo.

In the early years of teaching martial arts, I had a strong belief in tradition. The dojo was a place where respect and hard work were key, and I wanted my students to feel the weight of that responsibility. One afternoon, I was instructing a group of teenage students on a kata. They were doing well overall, but one student, in particular, kept making the same mistake, a small error that disrupted the flow of the form.

On his first mistake, I asked him to drop and give me ten pushups. He did so, though not without some grumbling under his breath. The second mistake came quickly after, and again I called for ten pushups. This time, there was a longer pause, a defiant look in his eye as he reluctantly went down. By the third mistake, he stood still, staring at me as if daring me to say it again.

"Pushups," I said firmly. But he didn't move.

There was a moment of tension in the air. The other students had paused their practice, and all eyes were on us. I could feel the weight of the moment—he wasn't going to do the pushups. He was tired, embarrassed, and frustrated, but so was I. I could sense I was on the verge of a power struggle, and if I insisted, I'd either have to physically enforce the pushups or somehow escalate the situation. Neither option seemed wise.

I stood there for a beat longer, weighing my options. I knew I was in an untenable position. Forcing him to comply would only erode my authority, not reinforce it. I had built this lesson around negative reinforcement—pushing them to be better by punishing mistakes. But now I was seeing that method blowup right in my face.

Instead of pushing further, I let out a breath, nodded, and calmly said, "Alright, let's do it together." There was a moment of surprise on the student's face.

I got down to the position and said, "We need to be in this together." We pumped out the push ups together. Then I did the kata with him and with the group, emphasizing the errors and working through the rough parts. Respect echoed in both directions.

I had swallowed my pride, but in doing so, I realized something crucial. Enforcing discipline shouldn't always be about punishment. I had been focusing so much on pointing out mistakes that I had forgotten to praise their successes and encourage their progress. By doing the push ups and the kata with him I demonstrated that I was invested in his success.

From that day on, I shifted my approach. Instead of fixating on what they were doing wrong, I started rewarding excellence. When a student executed a form flawlessly, I made sure the entire class knew it. When discipline was needed, I still enforced it, but in a way that focused on learning rather than punishment. And if I could show my own commitment to success, we'd work together as a team.

This allowed me never to be an evil enforcer, I became a brother in arms, a partner in crime. It's not quite Maciavellian. But it is in the sense that love is a better leader than fear.

The push ups became a tool for self-actualization rather than punishment, and the students began to push themselves harder—not because they were afraid of push ups, but because they were chasing the feeling of mastery. And I suffered along with them.

That teenage student? He never had to do another pushup for mistakes, but he did more of them voluntarily than anyone else in the class. As for myself, whenever I ask students to do pushups, we do them together; and I always do mine on my knuckles. I vowed never to demand something from a student that I couldn't, or wouldn't do myself.

Boxing

Around the same time, I began training at the Chino Boxing Club. Boxing was a completely different beast. It was raw, intense, and brutally honest. There was no room for error in the ring; every mistake was met with a punch that could be the end of the fight. My time at the Chino Boxing Club was both humbling and exhilarating. Boxing was one of my favorite forms of training. The thrill of stepping into the ring, the rush of adrenaline, and the satisfaction of landing a clean punch were unmatched.

Of course the fact that Bruce Lee favored boxing and even called his Jun Fan art Chinese Boxing expressed the significance he placed on boxing. As I started working on my fundamental skills with Coach Jerry, whose two sons also boxed at the gym and became lifelong friends, I was immediately attracted to the unforgiving need for power. If you had punching power, you could dominate in the ring. But boxing power and karate power are completely different.

Jerry believed that I had a future in the new sport of kickboxing. We worked on jab, cross, hook into back hook kick combinations because he thought it would be cool. But the opportunities for kickboxing didn't present themselves. There was no amateur kickboxing around and I wasn't old enough or in any position to try to go professional.

In the world of martial arts, karate and boxing represent two distinct approaches to combat. Karate emphasizes power and precision, with a focus on techniques that generate force from the ground up. The karateka's stance is a crucial element, providing a stable foundation from which to channel power through the body and into the opponent. The karate fighter believes he can take you out with one shot—one kick or punch to end the fight.

While this method works well for karate and karate fighting, it can be less effective against the mobile and agile boxer. The boxer's footwork and ability to close the distance quickly can disrupt the karateka's rhythm and make it difficult to land powerful strikes. The karateist may find themselves waiting in their stance for the perfect moment to strike, but by then, the boxer may have already unleashed a flurry of punches, slipping in and out of range with ease.

In contrast to karate, boxing emphasizes speed, agility, and power generated through body movement. While karate focuses on generating power from a stance, boxing emphasizes the use of body movement to enhance the force of punches. This dynamic approach to power is a key factor in the success of many great boxers and has made boxing one of the most popular and exciting combat sports in the world.

The boxer's ability to punch while their body is in motion enhances the force behind their strikes. The acceleration of the body adds to the power of the punch, creating a devastating force that can be delivered from various angles and targeted at multiple targets.

This is not to say that the karateist is inherently weaker, I would tell you that I can knock someone out using either method. It kind of reinforces itself, karateists should fight each other using karate, boxers stick to fighting boxers. Mixing the two against each other requires that one modifies their typical attack and defense to their opponent's skills and weaknesses; whatever style they may be.

Don "the Dragon" Wilson will tell you that he used his karate side and hook kicks to beat boxers in the ring. With 69 wins and 5 losses, 46 by knockout, he's the most winning kickboxer of all time.

Bill "Superfoot" Wallace, also a karate kickboxer used his lead left leg like a snake snapping and hooking his opponents.

The boxer can use their footwork to create angles and generate momentum, making their punches more difficult to defend against. Additionally, the boxer's ability to deliver punches from different angles and distances can keep their opponent guessing and off balance.

The fluid movements and rapid combinations of the boxer can overwhelm the karateka, who may struggle to adapt to the pace and intensity of the fight. The boxer's ability to bob and weave, combined with their inside punching techniques, can make it challenging for the karateka to land effective strikes.

But then there's the philosophy behind the fighter. The boxer knows he's fighting a war of attrition—although he could knock you out with one punch, his focus is the jab. Setting up the combinations. Taking the breath out of the body. Disrupting the strategy with headshots.

But one of the boxer's vulnerabilities comes with their tendency to lead attacks with their head forward. Their dependence on cover blocking can cause them to bring their gloves to their cheeks and tilt their head down and slightly forward, presenting an obvious target for a front or round kick right through their guard—causing the boxer to knock himself out, getting pummeled by his own hands.

I boxed with the Chino Boxing Club for two years, amassing a modest record of 1-1. My first match was a victory, a hard-fought battle that I won by decision. The second match didn't go as well. I took some heavy shots and ultimately lost. But even in defeat, there was a sense of accomplishment. Boxing tested my limits in ways I hadn't experienced before. It was a pure, unfiltered contest of skill, endurance, and willpower.

My second boxing match was a turning point, not just in the ring but in how I approached fighting altogether. I had trained hard, working on my technique, footwork, and combinations. Twice a week, I dedicated myself to karate, thinking it would keep me in shape for the fight. But as I was about to learn, conditioning for karate and conditioning for a boxing match were two very different things.

The first two rounds were a battle. My opponent and I were evenly matched, trading punches with intensity. I felt confident, my karate background giving me an edge in speed and timing. But by the end of the second round, a familiar feeling crept in: exhaustion. It hit me like a wall. My legs started to feel heavy, my breath came in ragged gasps, and my arms felt like rubber hoses filled with lead. No matter how hard I trained, I hadn't been conditioned enough for three full rounds of boxing.

You might think that three rounds is just 9 minutes. I can tell you that in the gym, I can easily do circuits of 10 rounds moving from heavy bag, speed bag, calisthenics and other drills for 45 minutes, easily. But add in the butterflies and adrenaline of a real match in the ring and three rounds of punching and fighting for your life is a slog.

As the third round started, it was clear I was in trouble. My hands were low, my reflexes dulled, and I was struggling to stay on my feet. I had entered pure survival mode. Every movement seemed like it took ten times the energy it should have, and every punch I threw felt slower, weaker.

In a moment of desperation, I threw a lead right cross, hoping it would land clean and shift the fight back in my

Copyright © 2025 Darryl Vidal

favor. My opponent, with more energy and awareness, simply sidestepped. I lunged too far forward and almost tumbled over the ropes. It was embarrassing, but worse, it was a reminder that I had nothing left in the tank. I was running on fumes.

I finished the fight. My opponent's conditioning had carried him through, while I could barely keep my gloves up by the final bell. The decision was unanimous—I had lost the fight. As disappointing as it was, that loss taught me a lesson I would never forget.

Conditioning is everything. No matter how skilled or experienced you are, without the stamina to back it up, you'll always be at a disadvantage. Someone out there will always train harder, push further, and be more prepared. That night, I learned to never take conditioning for granted again. From then on, I committed to training not just my technique but my endurance, knowing that in the ring, the better-conditioned fighter always has the edge.

Second point, karate by itself is not aerobic enough for endurance training. The karate student can do kata and drills endlessly, but in the ring would still gas by round 3. Endurance requires running, either on the road or the treadmill.

While my amateur boxing career may have been short-lived, the impact it had on my life was profound. The training methods and principles I learned during those years have remained with me and have become an integral part of my martial arts journey. My home gym training implements are: speed bag, heavy bag (Bob), double-end bag, dumb bells, Wing Chun dummy, pull-up rack.

Like Bruce Lee, I found that boxing training complimented my karate practice in numerous ways. The focus on speed, power, and agility was invaluable for developing my martial arts skills.

Skill development with each bag is a little different. Speed bag requires muscle elasticity and endurance. Shoulders are also built up. The Heavy bag training focuses on penetrating power. But also angles, combinations, footwork, speed and endurance. The double-end bag allows work on bobbing & weaving, blocking, angles while simulating attacks, providing a more aerobic session with the most footwork and ranging movement. These tools help to improve my hand-eye coordination, reflexes, and overall athleticism.

I learned to become proficient with the speed bag and the double-end bag. Both training implements you can hit as hard as you can. The double-end bag will even hit you back.

I particularly enjoyed bobbing and weaving drills, which helped me to improve my footwork and defensive skills. I also found it fascinating to learn how to balance objects on my nose, which is a great exercise for developing head-eye coordination.

In addition to the physical benefits, boxing also taught me valuable mental skills. The ability to shake off head shots and tighten up for body shots, hardens the body overall. The ability to push myself beyond my limits and persevere through challenges has been essential for achieving my goals.

While I may not have pursued a professional boxing career, my experiences in the sport have had a lasting impact on me. I can still balance odd things on my nose; sort of like a circus clown.

While I loved boxing, it began to have a noticeable impact on my karate, particularly in sparring. The rules of point system fighting in karate were very different from the full-contact nature of boxing. In karate, the goal was to score points by making controlled, precise strikes. However, after two years of boxing, I found it increasingly difficult to hold back. The intensity and aggression that boxing required didn't translate well to karate's more controlled environment.

I started getting disqualified in karate tournaments for excessive contact during sparring matches. My punches, conditioned by boxing, were too penetrating and often the combinations were too fast for the point system. It was frustrating because, on one hand, I was becoming a more formidable fighter, but on the other hand, my success in karate competitions was suffering.

Even today, if I catch you in a sparring match, make sure your mouthpiece is in place, because my right cross can be a little heavy.

Despite these challenges, I continued to dominate in kata competitions. Kata allowed me to express the full range of my martial arts training without the limitations imposed by the point system. My acrobatic kicks, Wing Chun, boxing, and even those early Escrima drills, gave my kata performances a unique flavor, blending fluidity, precision, and power in a way that set me apart from my peers.

The problem with boxing, which holds true to any type of martial arts training that includes striking to the

Copyright © 2025 Darryl Vidal

head, is the obvious problem with the long term effects of CTE - Chronic Traumatic Encephalopathy. Even during those two years of training, I can remember getting knocked out at least twice, and taking umpteen hard head-shots; where your head spins but you don't fall down.

This is why I don't encourage young kids to participate in sports with outright headstriking, like boxing, muay thai, and MMA. Even karate sparring and tae kwon do head kicking can be devastating.

Looking back, those years of cross-training were some of the most formative of my martial arts experience. Wrestling, Wing Chun, karate, boxing, and escrima each contributed something unique to my development as a martial artist.

Wrestling gave me the wherewithal to deal with the shoot and the takedown. Wing Chun taught me the importance of precision, efficiency, and direction of energy. Karate instilled in me a deep respect for tradition, form, and the role of the Sensei. Boxing, with its relentless focus on conditioning and mental toughness, pushed me to my limits and taught me the value of resilience and perseverance. And escrima, with its emphasis on fluidity and weaponry, provided the foundation for understanding oblique movement in combat.

Each discipline has its strengths and weaknesses, but together, they provide a comprehensive education in the martial arts. They also taught me that mastery was not about focusing on one thing to the exclusion of all else but about finding balance and harmony in a diverse range of skills.

As I continued my exploration, these early experiences in cross-training would become the bedrock of my martial arts philosophy. The lessons I learned in those years would shape my approach to training, teaching, and competition for decades to come.

Philosophically Speaking

Before going too deep into philosophies, I must qualify by saying these are my interpretations. I'm sure a PhD in any of these studies may find fault in my determinations, but at the risk of stepping on toes or mis-communicating notions, this chapter explores my own method of inquiry into Eastern and Western philosophies. The common thread through all this navel gazing mostly

Copyright © 2025 Darryl Vidal

comes back to natural law and the golden rule. We'll visit these in depth.

My exploration into the realms of religion and philosophy began in a setting that was familiar to many—Sunday mornings spent in a Protestant church. From a young age, my family adhered to a routine that included attending church services every week. The church was a central part of our lives, but not to the extent that it dominated our existence. We weren't the type to participate in Bible classes or extra fellowship groups.

Our faith was present, but it wasn't something that we lived and breathed every moment of the day. This approach allowed me to grow up with a solid grounding in Christian beliefs, but it also left room for curiosity and exploration.

The teachings of the church provided a moral framework, a sense of right and wrong, and a belief in a higher power. However, I wouldn't say that I was ever fully committed in the traditional sense. I absorbed the lessons, listened to the sermons, and participated in the rituals, but I always had a lingering sense of something more, something beyond the words spoken from the pulpit.

It wasn't that I doubted the existence of God or the importance of faith; rather, I sensed that there was a vast

Copyright © 2025 Darryl Vidal

and complex universe of ideas and beliefs waiting to be explored. This feeling became stronger as I moved into my teenage years, setting the stage for a lifelong quest to reconcile different strands of thought.

It was during high school that I first encountered the Tao Te Ching and the I Ching, two ancient texts that would profoundly shape my view of the world. I stumbled on to these texts as I explored Bruce Lee's Tao of Jeet Kune Do. It became clear to me that the Tao, and Taoism, was something much older and more significant than the teachings of a 20th century martial arts celebrity.

The Tao Te Ching, with its cryptic verses and paradoxical wisdom, introduced me to a way of thinking that was both alien and deeply resonant. It spoke of a fundamental force—Tao—that flowed through all things, a concept that seemed to align with the Christian idea of a divine presence in the universe. Yet didn't reinforce the ideas of a single Father, while the Son and the Holy Ghost held no parallels in the Tao Te Ching.

For myself as a young adult and college-age student, encountering both the Tao Te Ching and Christian teachings, the experience can be both enlightening and challenging as these two worldviews offer distinct ways of understanding life, purpose, and how to navigate the complexities of existence. At a fundamental level, both the Tao and Christianity teach valuable lessons about humility, balance, and living in harmony, but they take the individual down different paths to achieve those goals.

The Tao Te Ching with its focus on the Tao encourages students to let go of the need for control and embrace the natural flow of life. For someone in college, this idea of passivity can be a revelation or a detour, depending on one's perspective of God and heaven. In a world where striving, competition, and achievement are often celebrated, Taoism's message to surrender the ego and follow the natural order seems almost radical, yet in line with Jesus' humility and goodness.

It teaches that peace comes not from constant effort but from learning when to step back and let life unfold. On the other hand, Christianity offers a more structured, active approach to finding meaning in life. For a young adult navigating moral questions, personal identity, and relationships. It emphasizes love, justice, and humility in service to God. Christianity calls for a personal relationship with a loving God who is deeply interested in the individual's choices and future. For a college student, this idea of a personal, guiding force can offer comfort and direction in a time of uncertainty. But making these two meet in the middle presents the obvious conflicts.

While both traditions stress humility and letting go of pride, they differ in how they see the role of action. Taoism teaches that life's challenges should be met with flexibility and acceptance, often advocating for non-interference—whether that means not stressing about grades or avoiding conflicts. It can also be interpreted to let life lead you, and to fundamentally lose focus.

The lesson is to move with the current rather than fighting against it. A young person might learn to avoid burnout by practicing patience and self-compassion, trusting that not every problem needs to be solved immediately. It was clear that the martial artist could find solace and peace in the Taoist belief.

Christianity, by contrast, often emphasizes moral action and responsibility. It teaches that personal growth comes through choices and active engagement in the world—helping others, seeking justice, and growing closer to God through service and sacrifice. This might inspire one to take on leadership roles, get involved in social causes, or be more intentional about relationships with others, seeing these actions as part of a greater spiritual vision. These concepts are foreign to the Taoist expression which seems to abstract itself from daily life.

One of the biggest differences one might notice is in how each tradition views the divine. Taoism presents the Tao as an impersonal, abstract force, which can be freeing for someone who prefers to see life as a flow of events rather than something directed by a higher power. It encourages personal reflection and introspection, where peace is found by returning to a natural state of balance. This can appeal to persons who prefer a more philosophical, hands-off approach to spirituality.

On the other hand, Christianity offers a very personal understanding of God, where faith is a two-way relationship. The idea of God's grace and intervention provides a sense of security and hope, particularly during times of stress, loneliness, or doubt—a common experience in college life. The Christian belief in salvation through Jesus gives a clear narrative of purpose and redemption, which can provide direction when someone is trying to figure out their life path.

The I Ching, or Book of Changes, offered a system of divination that suggested a deep interconnectedness between human actions and the natural world, a concept that intrigued me and felt oddly familiar, even comforting.

The I Ching and Taoism are both ancient Chinese philosophies that share common roots, but they focus on different aspects of existence. The I Ching is centered on the balance and cyclical nature of life's forces. It presents life as a series of dynamic shifts between yin and yang, the two complementary forces that govern everything in the universe. The I Ching teaches that by observing the patterns of these changes, one can gain insight into how to act in harmony with the natural flow of events. It is deeply practical, offering guidance in navigating life's challenges by understanding the balance between opposing elements like light and dark, action and stillness, strength and softness.

Taoism, on the other hand, while also rooted in nature, goes beyond the balance of natural forces and seeks a deeper spiritual transcendence. The focus of Taoism is on the Tao itself—the underlying principle that governs the universe but remains beyond human comprehension. Taoism teaches that to live in accordance with the Tao, one must cultivate an understanding of the way things naturally are, while also striving to transcend personal desires, social constructs, and even the limits of intellectual thought. It calls for a more philosophical approach, where harmony with nature is not just about understanding balance but about becoming one with the Tao, the source of all life.

In the I Ching, the goal is to navigate the ups and downs of life by finding balance in the ever-changing flow of natural events. In Taoism, the goal is deeper—moving beyond life's changes to align oneself with the eternal Tao, living in harmony with the very essence of nature itself. Where the I Ching is grounded in the natural world and its cycles, Taoism invites one to go beyond, seeking unity with something more profound: the transcendent force that makes nature and life possible.

As I delved deeper into these texts, I began to see how Eastern philosophy could coexist with the Christianity of my upbringing. Rather than contradicting each other, these two traditions offered complementary perspectives on the same fundamental truths. Christianity provided a narrative of creation, sin, and redemption—a linear path with a clear beginning and end. In contrast, Taoism and the I Ching offered a more cyclical, harmonious view of existence, where opposites balanced each other and change was the only constant.

The idea that these philosophies could reinforce each other fascinated me. Christianity emphasized faith in God, while Taoism emphasized alignment with the Tao, or the natural way of things. What if these were simply two different ways of describing the same reality? Could God and the Tao be different facets of the same divine principle? These questions sparked a deep curiosity in me, one that would continue to grow as I expanded my philosophical horizons.

Throughout high school and into college, I continued to explore these ideas, seeking to understand how these seemingly disparate beliefs could be integrated. I read widely, trying to piece together a coherent worldview that encompassed both Eastern and Western thought. The more I read, the more I realized that both traditions sought to explain the same mysteries of existence—why we are here, what our purpose is, and how we should live our lives. Christianity spoke of salvation through faith and good works, while Taoism suggested that by living in harmony with the Tao, one could achieve a state of peace and contentment.

It became clear to me that these philosophies weren't in competition; they were complementary. Christianity's focus on the moral and spiritual guidance of an omnipotent God could be seen as providing a structure within which one could live in accordance with the Tao. In other words, Christian ethics could serve as a guide for aligning with the natural order described in Taoism. At the same time, the Taoist emphasis on balance and harmony could deepen one's understanding of Christian teachings, providing a more nuanced approach to living a life of faith.

As I grappled with these ideas, I began to see that the differences between Eastern and Western philosophies were more about perspective than substance. Where Christianity offered a more prescriptive approach to life, Taoism presented a descriptive one. Both, however, sought to guide individuals toward a life of virtue and fulfillment. This realization was both liberating and challenging, as it forced me to rethink some of the fundamental assumptions I had grown up with.

As I entered adulthood, my quest for understanding took on a new dimension with the introduction of science into my spiritual and philosophical explorations. I became fascinated by the mysteries of the universe, particularly through the lens of quantum physics. Here was a field of study that, like Eastern philosophy, embraced paradox and uncertainty. Quantum physics revealed a world that was far stranger and more interconnected than anything I had previously imagined. It suggested that reality was not as solid and fixed as it seemed, but rather a fluid, dynamic interplay of forces and energies.

The concept of reductionism became a tool for me to question others about their own beliefs. It offers the opportunity to explore wherein the soul exists. Why do we have a consciousness but a chair doesn't, and where in our bodies does this so-called consciousness exist?

This new understanding of the universe dovetailed with the spiritual concepts I had been exploring. Quantum physics, with its emphasis on the observer's role in shaping reality, seemed to echo the Taoist idea that perception and reality are deeply intertwined. The uncertainty principle, which states that certain pairs of physical properties cannot be known simultaneously with precision, reminded me of the Tao Te Ching's assertion that the Tao that can be spoken is not the eternal Tao; it's the first line of the text. Both pointed to a reality that was beyond full comprehension, a reality that could be sensed but not fully articulated.

I latched onto the concept of words being limited to man's assignment of meaning. Those words are interpreted

Copyright © 2025 Darryl Vidal

by man and similarly misinterpreted and even purposely miscommunicated.

Emergence offered yet another layer of perspective. To prove reductionism wasn't the final explanation. Where reductionism sought to explain the whole by dissecting it into its smallest parts, emergence proposed that complexity arises from the interactions within and between systems, producing phenomena greater than the sum of their parts.

A pod of orcas in a search and feeding mission, the neural interactions of the brain giving rise to consciousness, or the Constitution and the Bill of Rights—these are not merely the results of individual components but the products of intricate, interdependent relationships. It was a philosophy that resonated deeply with my psyche, uniting the insights of physics, spirituality, and personal growth into a coherent whole. Insisting that when sought, alternative realities and universes reveal themselves; without end.

As a young father, one of the greatest joys I found was sharing my passion for learning with my kids—and I wanted to nurture that inquisitive mind in each one of my children.

Reading was fundamental with all the kids as they grew. Nightly reading was something of a chore but these are moments we will keep all our lives; defining who we are in the world. Books like, "Where the wild things are," "Alexander and the Terrible, Horrible, No Good, Very Bad Day" have become stories that helped mold generations through scary and tough times. Even with my grandchildren now.

From an early age, I could tell Brad, my second son, had a sharp, logical mind—much like mine.

We did deeper reading like Moby Dick and of course Harry Potter. He was one of the only of ours that would read "chapter books" as they referred to any book without pictures.

It wasn't long before I decided to introduce him to some of the ideas that had captured my own imagination. One of the books that marked a turning point in that journey was Stephen Hawking's "A Brief History of Time."

Reading Hawking was a challenge, even for me. I'd always considered myself a logical thinker, but Einstein's theories of relativity, black holes, and quantum mechanics stretched my understanding in ways I hadn't expected.

Copyright © 2025 Darryl Vidal

Although a wonderful introductory book, Hawking has a penchant to jump to seemingly illogical conclusions without the explanation of how it was derived. Of course, any further inquiry in pursuit of said explanation requires a chapter in your college quantum physics text.

Still, I pushed myself to grasp the concepts, knowing that it would help me explain them in simpler terms for Brad and all my kids. I wanted him to see the beauty of the universe, not just as a collection of facts, but as a grand, intricate design—one that could be appreciated by anyone, without deep consideration.

Many evenings, I would sit with Brad, reading Hawking's words aloud, trying to distill the complexities of "Spin" and "Space/Time." I watched his eyes widen as we talked about the expanding universe, time dilation, and the possibility of other dimensions. I wondered if he was actually understanding it better than I was.

It wasn't just about the science for me, though—I always related what I read back to a bigger picture. How could the universe be so vast and mysterious without a Creator behind it? Where did God fit into Hawking's vision of the cosmos? Where do all the prayers go? Where have all the souls gone?

Copyright © 2025 Darryl Vidal

These weren't easy questions, but they were the ones I wanted all my children to wrestle with as they became adults. I never wanted them to feel like science and faith were at odds. Instead, I saw them as two sides of the same coin, each offering its own unique glimpse into the truth and the universe.

Bookworm

At that time in my life, I was becoming an avid reader. Not just science, but novels too. I picked up my first Tom Clancy novel, "The Cardinal of the Kremlin," in the airport on my first business trip, and that was it; I was hooked. I went back to the first book, "The Hunt for Red October" and read them in order through "Rainbow Six," with a smattering of many others in between. In fact I read "Hunt for Red October" at least three times and "Read Storm Rising" twice before I completed the series.

Never had I imagined that an author could make me feel like I'm in a Navy submarine hiding in shadows beneath the waves. Or in a sniper's den, waiting to take the six-hundred yard shot.

After I blew through the initial series of Jack Ryan stories I found other authors like Bond, Hagberg, Robinson,

Thor, Hunter and a cast of others that each brought a different flavor of perspective to the techno-thriller genre.

Sometimes the lines between them blurred—authors like Michael Crichton, with his deep dives into science fiction, or even John Grisham, whose legal thrillers sparked thoughts about justice and ethics. I'd read Jurassic Park and wondered how evolution and Chaos Theory fit into the divine plan, or finish a Clancy novel and think about the ethical implications of war and master diplomacy.

Darwin's "The Expression of the Emotions in Man and Animals" presented me with questions about creation that made me dig deeper into both science and theology.

There were nights when I'd have two books open at the same time—one fiction, the other non-fiction. A novel would capture my imagination while a science book would expand my understanding. They seemed to speak to one another, weaving a more complete picture of how the world worked and what our place in it was.

One of my favorite characters is Aloysius Pendergast. A fictional FBI agent of the Douglas Preston and Lincoln Child writing team. They wrote about Agent Pendergast's ability to use an ancient Tibetan meditation technique he used for solving crimes. Chongg Ran allows him to place himself in a deep state of pure concentration, where his mind could then combine all the facts and intuitions about a mystery and construct a multi-dimensional scene that could not only be analyzed but experienced. Through this memory crossing, Pendergast could reconstruct events from the past in his mind as if he were actually there, allowing him a unique forensic perspective. He would create this memory crossing in his mind using all historical and forensic data to recreate places, and even incidents that may have happened even years or centuries before.

After reading about Chongg Ran, I developed my own version of this technique and use it often to recall lost items and solve mysteries of the day. Of course it's much more simplistic than what might have been taught by the Tibetan monks, I'm sure my method shares in it's meditative approach to interacting within an experiential construct. The question is, can you create the construct in your mind detailed enough to interact with.

I have even helped some of my family members find lost items just by talking with them over the phone, asking questions about their day and time around the problem to be solved. I have been able to help others find keys or other

Copyright © 2025 Darryl Vidal

critical items just by questioning them, and building this memory crossing. Although I haven't solved any murders.

Reading works by physicists and philosophers like Paul Davies, and Michio Kaku, further expanded my yearning for understanding. These thinkers explored the implications of quantum mechanics, the nature of time, where God might fit into these inquiries, and the origins of the universe, often touching on questions that were as philosophical as they were scientific.

The more I read and thought about these ideas and concepts, the more I became convinced that science and spirituality were not only compatible but actually reinforce each other. Science provides the tools to explore and understand the physical universe, while spirituality offers a framework for interpreting and finding meaning to guide your soul and your psyche.

The idea of a God who created the universe was not contradicted by quantum physics; if anything, it was emboldened by it. The complexity and beauty of the universe, as revealed by science, became a testament to the power and wisdom of a divine creator. Nothing becomes more obvious than the fact that no evidence in science or physics contradicts or denies it.

Copyright © 2025 Darryl Vidal

These readings reinforced my time in the Eastern Sierras and my time fishing with my kids. A simple finger pointing to the edges of steep canyons and mountain lakes easily brought forth discussions about God and nature. I wish I could say they bore fruit. But that is their ideal to persue.

This synthesis of science and spirituality allowed me to develop a more nuanced and expansive view of God. No longer did I see God as merely a figure from religious texts; rather, I began to see God as the fundamental force behind the universe—the very fabric of reality itself.

This God is not distant or abstract but intimately connected to every aspect of existence, from the smallest subatomic particles to the vastness of the cosmos. It is a God that transcends the limitations of human understanding, yet is accessible through both faith and reason.

This realization brought me a profound sense of peace. It allowed me to reconcile the different strands of thought that had shaped my life—Christianity, Eastern philosophy, and science—into a coherent and fulfilling worldview. It is a worldview that embraces the mystery and complexity of existence, while still holding onto the belief

Copyright © 2025 Darryl Vidal

in a higher power that provides meaning and purpose to it all.

Even with this synthesis, my journey of exploration is far from complete. I continue to read, think, and question, constantly seeking to deepen my understanding of the universe and our place within it. I recognize that my beliefs will continue to evolve as I encounter new ideas and experiences. This ongoing quest is a central part of who I am. A reflection of my desire to live a life that is both thoughtful and spiritually rich.

In many ways, my approach to religion and philosophy mirrors my early experiences in church. Just as I didn't immerse myself fully in every aspect of Protestant life, I don't adhere rigidly to any one belief system now.

Instead, I draw from various traditions and ideas, piecing together a personal philosophy that resonates with me based on love of family and goodness. This approach allows me to remain open to new insights, while still holding onto the core beliefs that have guided me throughout my life.

Being very close to my mother, this spirituality became an important factor. She was raised Catholic, but my father raised us within the Protestant church. Her beliefs were strong and the fact that my wife was Jewish, and our children weren't baptised, marked her parenting as a failure in her mind.

Of course, nothing could be further from the truth. We were raised in a loving household and I always reflected to her that the importance of family and love were the key factors, and I think that was good enough to set her at peace. Especially once my own children bore her great-grandchildren. Their love was unequivocal leaving nothing more to bear out. There is nothing more satisfying than seeing your mother behold her great-grandchildren; of which she held four before she passed.

Ultimately, my religious and philosophical beliefs are rooted in a deep appreciation for the mystery of existence. I have come to accept that some questions may never be fully answered, that some aspects of reality may always remain beyond our comprehension. This uncertainty, far from being a source of anxiety, has become a source of wonder and inspiration. It reminds me that life is a journey of discovery, one that requires both humility and curiosity.

Enter C.S. Lewis

I first encountered Lewis through "Mere Christianity," a book that approached faith not with blind conviction but with rigorous logic and a profound respect for doubt. His oscillating views of Christianity, the devil, and the nature of humanity were like a bolt of lightning to my restless mind. Lewis did not ask me to abandon reason for faith; he invited me to explore the interplay between the two.

His portrayal of the devil in "The Screwtape Letters" revealed a cunning intelligence that preys on the mundane distractions of life, a subtle reminder of how easily we can drift from our ideals. It was not a red demon with horns but a reflection of my own procrastination, arrogance, and fears. Lewis's devil was a master linguist, twisting words and meanings to ensnare the unwary—a revelation that fascinated me as a student of both martial arts and language.

In reading The Screwtape Letters, I was struck by how brilliantly it presented the subtlety with which the devil approaches man. The devil's methods, as portrayed through the letters between Screwtape and Wormwood, reveal that our greatest battles with evil aren't fought in grand, obvious moments but in the small, daily struggles—through distractions, pride, and self-deception. The book made me realize that man's conflict with evil is often a slow erosion of character rather than a single act of rebellion. It challenged me to reflect on my own life, and how crucial it is to recognize the spiritual battles happening quietly within, and that every person is likely living this spiritual conundrum themselves.

Through Lewis, I began to see the Bible not as a rigid rulebook but as a work layered with metaphor, allegory, and poetry. Words, Lewis argued, shape our reality; they define and confine, liberate and illuminate. As a martial artist who communicated through movement and as a budding technologist fascinated by the logic of coding languages, this resonated deeply.

Lewis gave me a narrative—a story of a Creator who spoke the world into being, a Devil who sought to unravel it, and humanity's role as both actors and authors in this cosmic drama.

By embracing both the spiritual teachings of my youth and the scientific discoveries of modern times, I have found a way to navigate the complexities of life with a sense of purpose and meaning. My beliefs are not static; they are a living, evolving reflection of my ongoing search

Copyright © 2025 Darryl Vidal

for truth. And in this search, I have come to see that the true beauty of life lies not in having all the answers, but in the continuous pursuit of understanding, guided by both faith and reason.

Machiavelli and the 48 Laws of Power

As an adult, I made an effort to explore pure forms of philosophy, seeking to develop my own interpretations of the writings of the past masters. Machiavelli, Plato, Socrates and the 48 Laws of Power became essential texts in my intellectual journey. These works provided me with valuable insights that I have applied to my personal and professional life.

Machiavelli's The Prince offered a stark and controversial, but mostly misunderstood, perspective on the art of statesmanship and leadership. I particularly focus on his insights in understanding the realities of political life. His emphasis on the importance of power, fear, and cunning aligned with my own idealistic views of leadership, and management within the organization. Machiavelli's simplistic expressions of the lion and the fox, concepts that help rationalize behavior to achieve results, demonstrated a level of shameless pragmatism that I embrace.

In particular I gravitate to the concept of fear and love in organizational leadership. In most cases, love is a divine leadership method but fear works best most of the time and for most people.

Plato's The Republic provided a more idealistic vision of society, one based on reason, justice, and virtue. While I may not have fully embraced Plato's utopian vision, his ideas about the importance of education and the dangers of unchecked power resonated with me. Sometimes I would read, or listen to these texts, and find myself lost in my own thoughts. Their concepts trigger my own; a true exercise in self realization.

Additionally, as I delved into new endeavors, such as my own writings in the SciFi thriller MindCraft - the Educational Singularity - some of the concepts of utopia influenced my visions of futurism, artificial intelligence and leadership.

The 48 Laws of Power by Robert Greene offered a more practical guide to navigating the complexities of human relationships and power dynamics as well as providing an abridged version of these philosophers and other great leaders like Alexander the Great, Xerxes, Aristotle, Thoreau, Kissinger, and many many more. These laws, while often cynical, provided valuable insights into the strategies and tactics used by successful people throughout history.

I have found that the principles outlined in these works can be applied to various aspects of life, including business and personal relationships. In my own business dealings, I try to focus on competitive advantage and developing a trust-based relationship with partners and clients. This often requires recognition that they have the same motivations and self-interest; which becomes a focal point.

In my role as a martial arts instructor, I have also found the principles of these philosophical works to be relevant. As the sensei, the lion personality is preferred and respected. But in the sparring ring, especially regarding karate point-system fighting, the fox could be more cunning and successful.

Since I have been a "karate expert" all my adult life, I always maintain that it makes me a "really nice guy." Which reinforces the amiability that mitigates confrontations. Additionally, my busy lifestyle prevents me from being in places and situations which could precipitate confrontations. Basically, I don't go to bars and party like a madman.

Rule Breaker

If you've hung around with me any amount of time socially, you might know I'm a bit of a rule breaker. I don't want to say I'm an outright cheater, but I like to bend the rules whenever I can. If we're playing a friendly game, I'll typically do something, "not in the rulebook," to sway things my way. It's not that I'm a sociopath, but I do think it's entertaining to act out-of-the-box, as long as no one gets hurt—and there's no money involved.

As a flag football coach for my sons, we refined a playbook full of trick plays, along with standard plays that carried our teams undefeated for several seasons. I believe that an organized team will be a successful team. Flag football is about smart plays and sheer speed.

We had some bold plays, like pretending to be not lined-up and causing confusion in the formation, and as soon as the ref would blow the whistle we'd run the ball straight up the middle. Or splitting the receivers off to one side so you couldn't tell who was playing and who was on the sideline—then in the chaos, running the ball straight up the opposite sideline.

Probably one of the hardest games not to cheat at is golf. Golf is a pastime based on ethics and honesty. If you can't trust your playing partners in golf, then there can be no betting. Which is why I don't bet on golf. First of all, I'm not good enough—if I bet on my golf game, I would be a full-time money loser. Even my handicap is questionable.

Second, I don't like to "hit it as it lies." The pros get to play from pristine fairways and greens. They don't get dead spots, gopher holes and construction, unlike the average golfer. So I typically "adjust" my lie to be on a nice bed of fairway turf with a good stance. It's only fair.

I use the ground under repair loophole to get a good lie and a clear shot at the hole as much as possible—again, I don't play tournaments or for money.

If I do play for money, the pressure will surely get to me and I'll hit terrible shots. And besides that, I don't want to keep track of skins and such, so I won't know if I'm getting cheated.

Golf to me is a relaxing outing with friends or business partners, and I'll keep it at that. If you're one of those golfers that gets mad at their game, cussing and fussing, I'm not going to have fun with you. Only pros should get mad if they're not playing well. If it's not costing you big money, relax and take it all in stride.

Politics

In this writing I reflect on how my political views shaped the way I approached life, living, and personal responsibility. I don't want to marginalize half my potential audience by proclaiming the way my politics lean; but let's just say I lean toward morality, truth and love.

My beliefs are rooted in a desire for individual accountability, limited government, and the importance of preserving traditions that I felt were core to maintaining the values passed down through my family and community. This perspective wasn't about dismissing other viewpoints but rather about focusing on self-reliance and believing that people should have the freedom to forge their own paths without excessive interference and undue influence.

After high school, I was the only person I knew with any political bent. I became politically aware largely because my father was subtly political, and I wondered how his experiences as an immigrant influenced his thinking. I certainly agreed with his core values, and we would discuss

Copyright © 2025 Darryl Vidal

them in our times together. By the time I reached junior college, my political identity was already forming. I remember tuning in to the McLaughlin Group every Sunday morning for the only outlet for political discourse.

The lively debates and sharp commentary on current events captured my attention. I was drawn to the perspectives that resonated with the values I had learned from my parents—ideas around personal responsibility, strong national defense, and limited government.

The McLaughlin Group introduced me to political commentary in a way that sparked a deeper interest in the broader political movement. While my peers might have been focused on sports or other normal kid activities, I was engrossed in this show, forming my opinions on the role of government and society. It became a ritual of sorts, shaping my understanding of the politics and solidifying the tenets I would live by throughout my adult life.

I particularly related to traditionalists like Mort Kondracke, Fred Barnes, and of course, John McLaughlin himself. Their perspectives resonated deeply with the values I had grown up with—emphasizing personal responsibility, hard work, and patriotism.

Copyright © 2025 Darryl Vidal

Of course, Elenor Clift was the reliable liberal viewpoint they all countered, and ganged up on.

Watching them debate on the McLaughlin Group provided examples of how one's values and morals could form the basis of a political stance, but a way of viewing the world and one's role within it.

Mort Kondracke often brought a measured approach to the discussions, advocating for a pragmatic conservatism that emphasized maintaining the strength of America's institutions while being cautious of sweeping reforms. I appreciated how he would balance his support for fiscal responsibility with a recognition that some government interventions were necessary to maintain societal stability.

Fred Barnes, on the other hand, was often more direct in his defense of limited government and lower taxes, arguing that overregulation stifled the entrepreneurial spirit. His commentary often emphasized the importance of economic freedom and the idea that individuals, not the government, should be the ones driving economic progress. I found myself agreeing with Barnes on this, as I too believed that people should have the freedom to pursue success without undue government interference.

And then there was John McLaughlin, whose sharp wit and commanding presence guided the panel's discussions. McLaughlin was unafraid to challenge liberal viewpoints and was a proponent of strong national defense and traditional values. His ability to cut through the noise and get to the core of an issue was something I admired.

Whether he was debating the need for military strength during the Cold War or stressing the importance of upholding moral standards in society, McLaughlin's convictions mirrored the principles I was developing at the time.

I always loved to close a meeting or discussion with a concise answer to the question at hand, and a final, "Bye Bye!"

These figures shaped my early understanding of my own philosophical construct. Through their debates, I saw how my own view was not just about resisting change for the sake of tradition, but about preserving the core values that I believed made society strong—individual liberty, personal responsibility, and a deep respect for institutions like the family, the military, and country.

In martial arts, just as in life, I saw the value in discipline, earning what you worked for, and respecting authority—not because it was imposed, but because it was deserved.

I drew parallels between my training and my political philosophy: just as in the dojo, where hard work, respect, and focus led to progress, I felt that in society, individuals thrive when they're empowered to take control of their own futures.

These ideas of perseverance, personal growth, and accountability intertwined with my worldview, influencing how I navigated both my career and personal life. They became guiding principles, shaping not just my outlook on politics, but on how I interacted with others and set the course for my own exploration and transcendence.

Lessons from Sensei

The following chapters are a reprise of a speech that I had delivered several times to my students and martial arts gatherings.

Anger

When I was still a brown belt, during a class with Sensei Rosas, I was often paired with lower-belt students to demonstrate sparring techniques. One day, during a sparring session, a particularly aggressive student challenged me in front of the entire class. He taunted me, dancing back and forth, sticking his chin out as if daring me to hit him. At the time, we referred to this student as "hyperactive," but in today's terms, he would likely be described as being "on the spectrum." Looking back, I realize the idea of "teaching him a lesson" was misguided from the start.

Despite being older and more experienced, I allowed myself to be provoked by his relentless taunts. Instead of staying calm and composed, I gave in to a moment of anger. Stepping forward, I threw a hard right cross that landed squarely below his left eye, sending him to the ground, clutching his cheek. It wasn't a proud moment, even though I had succeeded in silencing his provocations.

Sensei Rosas immediately called a halt to the sparring session. He didn't say a word, but his glare spoke volumes. The lesson was over for the day. Later, he pulled me aside and explained that, while it was important to defend oneself, it was equally important to do so with control and restraint. He emphasized that maintaining a calm and focused mind is essential, even when provoked. More importantly, I was being presented as an advocate, a model. This behavior was not acceptable. That was it.

His words were a reminder that martial arts isn't just about physical strength or skill but about mastering one's anger and emotions.

I was deeply embarrassed and ashamed of my actions. I had allowed my anger to take control and had set a poor example for the other students. Sensei Rosas' quiet rebuke was a harsh but necessary lesson. That day, I learned that being a martial artist goes beyond technique—it requires mental focus and emotional control. It was a lesson that stayed with me and shaped how I would approach training from that point forward.

Ambition - The Pursuit of the Black Belt

Under the watchful eye of Sensei Rosas, I developed a deep-seated ambition to achieve the rank of Sho Dan (Black Belt). This was not merely a goal; it was a calling, a testament to my dedication to the art of karate. The path to black belt was a long and arduous one, requiring years of tireless training, unwavering commitment, and relentless perseverance.

This is not something that one simply sets his mind to and then pursues relentlessly. In actuality, it's something done almost inconsequentially; without significant thought or planning.

I always say, I never set out to be a Grandmaster, I simply ended up here. It's much the same way for Sho Dan (first degree black belt). You don't think about pursuit, or greatness. You just go to class each night and train as prescribed. The trick is to keep coming back and making forward progress. Even if you're not feeling up to it or running late. You still make it to class and give it your best.

Each belt test comes along, presents its challenges, and becomes your next conquest. There's not necessarily as much blood and sweat as advertised. It's really more about being there. Being present, and performing. But because of the interest and ambition, the training takes on a life of its own. Outside of class. Even in your daily thoughts and feelings.

I dedicated countless hours to honing my skills, practicing techniques until my muscles ached and my mind exhausted. I participated in tournaments, testing my abilities against other martial artists and pushing myself to new limits. I also assisted Sensei Rosas in teaching classes, sharing my knowledge and experience with younger students.

With limited funds but a surplus of my dad's garage full of random items, I transformed our garage into a makeshift workout gym. My first project was a heavy punching bag, which I crafted by hand-stitching heavy canvas with wax string and upholstery needles.

I went to the High School woodshop and collected sawdust from the dumpster to fill the heavy bag. Using the sawdust and a bunch of old blankets, the large punching bag was the centerpoint of my new gym. The result was a sturdy, homemade training tool that could withstand the most punishing blows, although a puff of sawdust would leak out of the seams with each heavy kick.

I then created focus pads. Basically, rectangular pillows with finger and wrist straps used for punching and karate drills. Only problem with these is you need a partner, who knows what they're doing.

Next, I turned my attention to the makiwara, a traditional Japanese striking pad. Using the sewing machine and heavy-duty needles and thread, I carefully constructed smaller versions of the makiwara, providing me with additional targets for my training. It mixed them up with different stuffing, rice for a softer makiwara, sand for a harder one.

While I couldn't afford a commercial speed bag mount, I improvised by cutting the circular top from thick particle board and creating mounting brackets using spare angle iron. With a little ingenuity and elbow grease, I had a functional speed bag setup that allowed me to work on my hand-eye coordination and reflexes. The only things I had to buy were the swivel and the bag itself. Unfortunately, you learn quickly that the bag size and the swivel are super important.

So, the ball bearing swivel and the custom Cleto Reyes peanut bag made of top quality leather, and balanced like a top, made up the final more costly components of the setup.

My homemade boxing gym was a testament to my resourcefulness and dedication. It provided me with a space to train on my own terms, without the constraints of expensive equipment or crowded gyms (which weren't really things at the time}. Through countless hours of practice and perseverance, I honed my karate and boxing skills and prepared myself for the ultimate challenge.

The journey to black belt was not without its risks and diversions. There were times when I doubted my abilities, when the physical and mental demands seemed overwhelming. But I refused to give up. I drew strength from my passion for karate and my determination to succeed.

Additionally, the weekly karate tournaments kept me focused on the ultimate goal of the black belt. Even though I was beating lower belts and other brown belts consistently both in kata and kumite, there were still many black belts walking around, competing, and winning. These are the people I'm gonna have to compete with once I get my Sho Dan I often recognized. These guys were tough, most of them bigger than me, and much more experienced in face-contact kumite.

As I ascended the ranks, the requirements for the Sho Dan test seemed to multiply. It felt like every time I thought I had mastered one aspect of the curriculum, another layer of complexity was added. The pressure to meet these ever-evolving standards was immense, and at times, it felt like Sensei was just adding things indiscriminately to make it more difficult.

There were moments when I questioned whether the pursuit of black belt was truly worth the effort. The physical and mental demands were exhausting, and the constant pressure to perform at a high level was taking a toll on me. I even considered quitting after a particularly difficult training session when additional requirements were mentioned. I thought of quitting karate altogether and focusing on boxing, a sport that I had always been interested in.

However, as I reflected on my path in karate, I realized that it was more than just a martial art; it was a way of life. Karate had taught me discipline, perseverance, and the importance of setting and achieving goals. Giving up would mean betraying the values that I had come to cherish. I came to the realization that I would probably always be a martial artist, for the rest of my life.

Ultimately, I decided to press on with my training. I understood that the challenges I faced were a natural part of the road to black belt. That I was already heavily invested in the undertaking and walking away would be like walking away from a philosophy and belief system to guide my mind and soul. By overcoming these obstacles, I would become a stronger and more resilient martial artist.

The Sho Dan test was an ordeal—a true test of my physical and mental fortitude. It lasted for several hours, covering every aspect of the curriculum, from basic techniques and katas, to the compulsory katas, weaponry, advanced self-defense techniques ending with sparring.

When I finally achieved my black belt, it was a moment of immense pride and satisfaction. I had achieved a goal that I had worked towards for many years. But more importantly, I had learned valuable lessons about perseverance and the power of the human spirit. The black belt was not merely a symbol of my martial arts accomplishments; it was a testament to my character and my ability to overcome challenges.

Looking back 40 years later, quitting before black belt would have been the biggest mistake of my life—especially as far as the Karate Kid goes.

Sho Dan Test

The success I achieved in kata and sparring competitions played a crucial role in preparing me for the ultimate test of my martial arts endeavor—my black belt test, scheduled for June 6, 1981. This significant event came shortly after graduating from high school and represented the culmination of four years of intense training and dedication. My black belt test was a four-hour trial, designed to rigorously assess all the foundational movements, stances, strikes and kicks, katas, self-defense techniques and weapons I had mastered.

It was a comprehensive demonstration of everything I had learned, pushing me to showcase my skills at the highest level.

The panel of judges for this pivotal moment included some of the most respected black belts in the martial arts community, many of whom had overseen my progression through the colored belts. Among them were legendary figures like Dan Guzman, Joe Rosas' instructor, along with Dave Torres, George Franco, Rudy Cordero, Arturo Ruiz, Richard Garcia, Mark Sells, and "Fast" Eddie Romero. Their presence underscored the seriousness of the test and the high standards I was expected to meet.

The sparring portion of the test was particularly intense. At one point, a sparring partner came on too aggressively; should I tell you that he tried to show me up—show that I wasn't ready? I probably wouldn't normally interpret it that way as the sparring in a black belt test is always intense.

In reality it was a close friend. We had come up through the ranks together. We even tested together all the way up to brown belt. But during our brown belt tenure, we both had life occurring. I was graduating from high school, had been boxing and cross-training with others and recently had overcome the mental lapse of possibly quitting in frustration.

He was also amidst a break. He was dealing with his own issues—I'm telling you that this year as a brown belt is a slog.

I ended my break from karate with a personal goal to test for Black Belt before leaving for the Philippines in the Summer of 1981. I told Sensei Rosas that I would be leaving for three months and requested to be tested beforehand. So my test was moved up to June of 1981, while my karate buddy was still on his hiatus.

All those years of training and testing together, it was always assumed we would test for Sho Dan together. So while we both took a short break, I came back first and moved the test date closer, and accelerated the training and intensity of my preparation. Since he wasn't around, he didn't find out that I was testing until the weekend of the actual test. It would be impossible to test together.

In fact, he wasn't even invited to the test, since he hadn't been attending class for almost half a year.

So, in the third hour of my black belt test, he showed up—in street clothes. He was incensed, he felt slighted. He felt as if I intentionally betrayed him by testing alone early. This is what I believe as we've never discussed it. I may be wrong but it sure felt that way. But it really was just a matter of happenstance. I came back—he wasn't around.

He asked to borrow someone else's gi so he could join the line of brown and black belts I would have to fight for the final Kumite portion of the test.

I always joke that black belt tests are kind of like a gang initiation. A line of senior belts take turns for 2 minutes of all-out beat down. You must show you can protect yourself from getting pummelled by a bunch of senior belts. By the fourth or fifth fight, the candidate is typically beaten to exhaustion. It's really a test of heart—that's how we rationalize it, anyway.

So my karate buddy was intent to show that I wasn't ready. He came at me hard to prove his point. Kicking and punching for effect. Trying to show my weakness—dare I say it? Trying to hurt me. But I was in top form.

He ended up with a broken jaw and severe lacerations to the upper lip. The gi that he had borrowed was covered in blood. The injury required the jaw to be wired and the lip to be stitched both internally and externally, a stark reminder of the physical demands and risks involved in martial arts.

This dramatic incident highlighted the seriousness of the test and the need for both skill and control in martial arts practice—and the importance of a mouthpiece.

The point of this lesson on ambition. Set your sites, and nothing can get in your way.

Excellence

Sensei Rosas was a demanding instructor who insisted on excellence in everything we did. He drilled us on the fundamentals, demanding precision and accuracy in our technique. He taught us the importance of proper stance, power generation, and timing.

I quickly realized that mastering the basics was essential for achieving higher levels of proficiency. By focusing on the fundamentals, I was able to develop a solid foundation that would serve me well throughout my martial arts career.

Even last night in class, as I prepared several green belt for their brown belt test, we went back to fundamentals. Stance, balance, focus, power; the qualities of the skilled martial artist.

Sensei Rosas also emphasized the importance of teaching others. Beginning as a brown belt, and then in preparation for black belt, I was expected to assist in teaching classes and to serve as a role model for younger students. This experience taught me the value of giving back to the community and helping others to achieve their goals.

It is quickly realized, when teaching someone else, that you have to know, not only what you are doing, but why. If you don't know why, you will at best look silly, but at worst, lose credibility. There's nothing worse than trying to explain some strange movement, when you don't know why you're doing it.

If you don't even know exactly what you're teaching, you're going to have to ask someone else, risking teaching it wrong—this is a cardinal sin in karate instruction.

By demanding excellence from his students, Sensei Rosas helped us to reach our full potential. He pushed us beyond our limits, challenging us to strive for greatness.

His unwavering belief in us inspired us to achieve things that we never thought possible.

From this lesson I came to embrace the idea that by demanding excellence, we help others achieve excellence.

Community

Sensei Rosas taught through the Chino Parks and Recreation department. This was a unique approach that set his program apart from many other martial arts schools. By teaching through a recreation-based organization, Sensei Rosas was able to make martial arts accessible to a wider range of people.

I initially had some reservations about training with the recreation department karate class. It was like in the Karate Kid when Daniel's mom says, "You took karate." Daniel retorts, "Not at the Y, a real karate school." Referring to the YMCA—another community-based organization.

I had always imagined myself training in a traditional dojo with a more austere atmosphere. However, I soon realized that the true dojo was not a physical place, but rather the learning environment created by the instructor and the students.

Sensei Rosas fostered a strong sense of community among his students. We trained together, supported each other, and celebrated our successes. We became more than just classmates; we became a family.

By teaching through the community, Sensei Rosas was able to make a positive impact on the lives of hundreds of thousands of people. He helped to build self-esteem, promote physical fitness, and teach valuable life lessons. His commitment to his community was an inspiration to me and to many others.

Discovered!

The Pursuit of Hollywood and Vice Versa

My dream of becoming a martial arts movie star was fueled by my early successes in karate competitions. I had developed my own kata that incorporated explosive jumping and spinning kicks, techniques that often left my opponents bewildered and defeated. My dominance in both kata and kumite competitions convinced me that I had the talent and drive to achieve similar fame.

However, while I had the martial arts skills, I lacked the knowledge and experience to break into the film industry. I wasn't one of those kids whose parents wanted stardom for their children.

If you met one of them you'd know. They would drive to Hollywood several times a week for auditions and meetings with their agents. They'd pay hundreds of dollars for headshots, singing and acting lessons. I had neither the money or wherewithal to take on this effort.

In my early college years, I decided to take an acting class, believing it might be the key to unlocking a career in show business. The class itself was an exciting experience—it provided me with some exposure to the stage and taught me basic performance techniques. However, what it didn't offer was any insight into the real-world aspects of the acting profession. I found myself at a loss when it came to understanding how to take the next step: How do I get an audition? How did I find an agent? What did it take to stand out in Hollywood, a place filled with aspiring actors all fighting for a shot?

Despite the lack of practical guidance, my dream of becoming a martial arts movie star never faded. I had grown up watching the legendary Bruce Lee, and in my mind, I knew I had the talent and passion to make it in that world. But simply being talented wasn't enough. As I began to understand the magnitude of the competition, I realized I needed to learn the ins and outs of the industry—something my acting class alone couldn't provide.

This was decades before you could Google "How to get into show business." The best we had was to go out to Hollywood and get your hands on the show business rags like Variety, the Hollywood Reporter, and Backstage. But even that was more than I could commit to while working and going to junior college. Basically, I realized I did not have the means or ambition or parents to do this the regular way.

Determined, I started researching everything I could about the film industry. I devoured books and articles from the library, studied the careers of my martial arts idols like Bruce Lee, Jackie Chan, and other martial arts pioneers that were breaking into show business.

I saw that a lot of the Chinese Kung Fu movies were produced by the Shaw Brother's and Golden Harvest films. Both Chinese companies that I had no way of contacting in the 1980s.

Copyright © 2025 Darryl Vidal

What became clear was that success in Hollywood required more than just skill in front of the camera—it was about networking, constantly auditioning, and building relationships with industry professionals. Still, even with this new understanding, I found it difficult to even take the first step. The industry was tough, and while my passion remained strong, navigating its maze of closed doors and unspoken rules was a challenge I couldn't understand.

Another thing I didn't understand at the time was that Hollywood was still dominated by white people. People of color, and Asians for the most part, were practically non-existent in Hollywood. Pat Morita was definitely the exception.

A Hollywood Story

My journey toward becoming a martial arts movie personality (I refuse to say "star") took an unexpected turn at a karate tournament in Los Angeles. It was Juan Larios' 1983 Fiestas Open Karate Championship at Southgate HS. I had just won the kata competition. Unbeknownst to me, the director of the iconic film "Rocky" and his assistant were in attendance, scouting for talent for a new project.

Even this bit of trivia, the event and location, was lost on me for over 30 years. It wasn't until Facebook came about that one of many unknown "friends" told me that he was there when the meeting happened.

As I sat on the gym floor, putting on my foot gear and getting ready for the kumite competition. I was approached by the director's assistant Randy Sabusawa. To my astonishment, he asked me if I would be interested in being in a movie. I was taken aback by the unexpected opportunity, but I quickly recovered and said, "Of Course!" and asked for more details.

Randy introduced me to a short middle-aged gentleman in street clothes and introduced him as John Avildsen, the director of Rocky. I stood there astonished but skeptical as he handed me a piece of paper with contact information and instructions to call the number on Monday morning.

So I did. He told me to come to the soundstage at one of the studios in Burbank. I was filled with excitement and disbelief. Could this be a real opportunity to break into the film industry? The opportunity that had been so elusive for all these years fell right into my lap.

My father would echo an adage repeated at my eighth grade graduation ceremony. "Success is the crossroads of preparation and opportunity. You can prepare all your life, but without the opportunity, you cannot be successful. Alternately, you can have the opportunity, fall into your lap, but if you're not prepared…"

So it wasn't pure luck, I was prepared. I had been preparing for years. The opportunity arose because I was attending karate tournaments regularly, and winning. So the whole Hollywood story is about preparation, opportunity, and luck.

After years of wondering how I would ever get a break and get into a martial arts film may have worked the "old fashioned" way; getting discovered. It was a true Hollywood story as I would say in interview after interview.

I left the tournament that day with a sense of exhilaration and anticipation. I couldn't wait to find out more about the movie project and the role I might be auditioning for. The thought of appearing on screen, alongside famous actors and actresses, was both thrilling and intimidating. I cautioned myself of being too confident—this could turn out to be nothing.

My parents were skeptical—this never happened in real life. But there was no debate, I would show up at the studio as requested. I had nothing to lose—except gas money.

In my conversations with John and Randy, I had asked, "So what's the name of the movie?" John said, "The working title is the Karate Kid." I stifled a giggle and tried to wipe the stupid grin off my face, and I thought, only to myself, that's a dumb name for a movie. Luckily, I was smart enough not to say that outloud, although I swear I must have heard several others voice the same opinion over the years.

As I waited for Monday to arrive, I began to prepare for the audition. I had no idea what they had in mind, so I couldn't practice acting or doing anything but my kata that they had watched me perform at the tournament.

When I arrived at the soundstage the next morning, Randy along with John Avildsen, I was introduced to many of the cast and crew. To my surprise, I recognized Pat Johnson, a renowned stunt coordinator and martial arts expert who played a gangster-type in Enter the Dragon. Things started to get real.

Copyright © 2025 Darryl Vidal

As we walked across the backlot, a Rolls Royce drove up and parked near one of the office trailers. It was there that I was introduced to the world renown Jerry Weintraub, movie producer extraordinaire. Now I knew this was legit—as if being checked in at the studio gate wasn't enough.

I also met Ralph Macchio, the young actor who had been cast in the lead role of Daniel Webber. It would be changed to Daniel LaRusso later, to give him a more New Jersey Italian heritage. Of course I didn't know who Ralph was at the time. But I held to my politeness and stuck to the role of Hollywood neophyte and played it cool. I didn't want to come across too excited but I had to balance that with being low key. The last thing I wanted was to come across as arrogant or condescending, since it would seem I was the only one besides Pat Johnson that really knew karate.

Another familiar face was Pat Morita, the veteran actor who would be playing the role of Mr. Miyagi. We made an immediate connection because back in the eighties, we found a commonality in our Asian backgrounds. Pat and I immediately hit it off. I recall him always joking and acting silly. He was a genuinely funny and happy guy.

He was happy to meet me and started off with many of his one-liners that I wish I could recall accurately. They basically rolled off his tongue non-stop—often saucy and explicit as was the basis of his comedy.

Working with Pat Morita is a truly inspiring memory. He was a kind and generous man who shared his wisdom and experience with the younger cast members.

In my first meeting with them at the rehearsal stages, I was asked to perform my kata for the crowd. It was a side of a sound stage with gymnasium-style seat benches along one wall. The area in front of the stands was covered with a mat for gymnastics or stunt-work—perfect for doing karate.

John called me over and introduced me to the crowd gathered in the stands and asked me to do that kata I did at the tournament. It was my moment. This would be the audition. The crowd was polite as I stepped up to the middle of the ring and performed my kata as if I were in competition.

I debated whether or not to describe the kata here. I'm not sure I can think of anything more boring than reading a description of a kata—no matter how exciting it might be.

Let me just say that every move you see me do in the Karate Kid, except for the crane kick, is in my kata.

I would start with a jumping Russian-split kick, landing and then turning into a high, slow-motion knife-edge kick with the right leg. Then some strikes to the left side followed by a back-hook into a drop-down back sweep. After several strikes and kicks that orient me facing forward, I would end with back hook, jumping back hook, into drop down back sweep. Then into a high front kick and drop down into a split. Lots of spinning and jumping.

The most memorable moves from the Karate Kid fight with Johnny Lawrence are the triple tornado kicks, correctly called jumping outside inside crescent kicks, and of course the jump back spin, which Johnny evades and drops me spectacularly with a kick to the head, which dispatches me hard to the floor. Quite a spectacle of a kata!

The crowd buzzed as I finished. I can recall Ralph saying, "Dynamite," good thing you're not an actor, I'd lose my part."

Ralph and I didn't have much interaction in the Summer of 1983 as most of my rehearsal time was spent with the Cobra Kai actors, training and doing choreography with Pat Johnson.

I recall following Pat Johnson into the soundstage and meeting all the Cobra Kai members. There was Billy Zabka, Tony O'Dell, Rob Garrison, Ron Thomas and Chad McQueen. I was most impressed by Chad as his father was the movie star Steve McQueen, whom I also knew had trained with Bruce Lee.

It was in these early rehearsals that I met Fumio Demura and Gerald Okumura. They were on set to meet with John Avildsen and writer Robert Mark Kamen to audition for the Miyagi character as well as other stunt roles they needed to cast.

These martial artists were already legends well known to me at the time. Pat Johnson had appeared in my favorite martial arts film Enter the Dragon. Fumio Demura was well known for his demonstrations at the famed Japanese Deer Park in Buena Park and several books and magazine spotlights. Gerald Okamura had appeared in Kung Fu and the Octagon.

Of the Cobra Kai actors, Ron Thomas and I began to come together and joke around because I had suspected that he was also a trained martial artist like myself. Billy Zabka also became a friend during these rehearsals and we spent a

Copyright © 2025 Darryl Vidal

lot of time training and practicing our choreographed semi-final fight.

Billy was very athletic, a former wrestler, and we began to work closely together, working on creating a realistic depiction of a karate point-system fight. He would go on to use much of our training together in his other fight sequences.

Years later, while recalling those early years, Billy recounted to me that I had asked him if he could take a shot to the body during our sequence to help it look more realistic. Although initially unsure, he said,"Sure, I can take it."

As it happened, I pounded on him several times during our sequences together, but he just took the hits in stride realizing that I wasn't hitting him with a full follow through, and that he was cool with the contact.

We trained as a cohesive dojo with Pat Johnson and the Cobra Kai team for several weeks in the Summer of 1983 and although the training was legitimate karate drills and practice, we never sparred; actors aren't allowed to spar to prevent from getting injured.

Although I didn't realize it at the time, separating the Cobra Kai students from Ralph and Pat's training was brilliant. It allowed the Cobras to develop a team dynamic and Pat and Ralph to train in isolation—even slightly encouraging the Cobras to dislike Ralph.

The Crane Technique

During rehearsals for the second week, Director John Avildsen, writer Robert Mark Kamen and Pat Johnson approached me about another part for the movie. They must have been satisfied with my raw abilities and my can-do attitude. This would be a moment that would transcend all my dreams and fantasies about martial arts and movie stardom. Who would know decades later that this one event would be the moment I would never live down—yet for most people, I would never be recognized for—even as I write this today (2025).

Robert explained to me that Daniel, with one leg injured during the tournament, would be forced to do a jumping kick technique while standing with the injured leg raised. To support this premise in the storyline, Miyagi would be seen performing the technique while standing atop a stump during a beach scene as if it were some mystical ancient fighting method.

It was something that was portrayed in the kung fu movies in a very fantastic way. With kung fu men standing and hopping from tree branches or scaffolds in incredible demonstrations of balance and power.

The "Crane Technique" would be performed with one leg raised and arms outstretched to the side like a large bird. That was the way it was described to me by writer Robert Kamen. He would tell me later that he believed the move to be almost impossible in real life—which it was in the exact description.

The technique was described as, "with the arms outstretched like a great bird, jumping from the one-legged stance, kicking with the leg, and then landing with the same leg."

My first instinct was to say to John and Robert, "why would you ever do that? That wouldn't work." The answer came quickly, "because it's the crane technique." I quickly learned to keep my mouth shut and do what they wanted.

I knew in my mind that the mechanics of the crane technique wouldn't work and I was doubtful. They gave me some practice time to work out the bugs on the technique. After practicing what they described I struggled with the idea of jumping from my right leg (base) and then landing with it.

In karate circles it was typical to do what we called a "double-jump" kick starting with one leg chambered and then kicking with the base leg, however, this double-jump kick allowed you to land on the raised leg.

This was also called a "pump-fake" kick using the raised knee chamber as a fake, and then jumping into the second front kick, launching forward and landing on the formerly raised leg.

In fact, we used to practice this double-jump kick, by raising the leg, which was the initial fake kick, jumping into the front kick, and landing with the kicking leg still chambered. Then jumping into the next front kick from this position. Not only was it good exercise but you could then do the double-jump from either side, while moving toward your opponent.

But this request was much different, not only did they want me to jump, kick, and land with the same leg, but they wanted me to be atop a 12" round stump. The hands outstretched to the side were inconsequential at this point as none of it seemed realistic anymore. It was just the

Copyright © 2025 Darryl Vidal

"crane technique." No other explanation required in Hollywood.

I went over to Ron while the Cobra Kai team was on break and showed him what they wanted. He was skeptical as we were both very familiar with the double-jump style kick. I thought it would be impossible without taking a running start. It would not work on top of a stump without some modification.

I decided that the best thing to do was convince them that a double-jump kick would work. I showed them how I could start with a Kenpo Karate cat-stance, and then raise the leg into the knee up position, then I did a double-jump kick and landed in the same spot with the opposite leg, then quickly switched back to the cat-stance, low.

This kick allowed for me to raise one leg, jump and kick with the other leg, and then land on the formerly raised leg. This did not meet the exact technique they had described but after some discussion and demonstration, they agreed the double-jump kick would work.

After watching me practice it several times, the director and the writer said, "the kick looks great, but you've got to do something with your hands."

So I started in the cat stance with my hands in a Wing Chun style (hands open in a low forward guard). Then I would lower myself down, then rise up in a tall one-knee-up position with my arms fully outstretched to the sides; fingers angled down like the feathers of a great crane. Then, explode the double-jump kick and land back in the cat stance (switching back to the original stance in the next moment). They liked it. The move was formally dubbed the Crane Technique. I didn't think much of it at the time because to me, it was a silly version of the same old double-jump kick.

Next we had to figure out how to practice on top of a stump or post. This was totally lost on me as the kung fu movies always depicted them on top of branch-like sticks with the experts jumping from stick to stick.

As I dug for more details Pat told me they were going to cut a telephone pole and bury them vertically in the sand as if they were pilings from an old broken-down pier. That made more sense. I imagined a telephone pole to be about 12" around. That, I could handle.

In order to simulate the stump, I took a walk over to the studio cafeteria at lunch and brought back a few paper plates. I placed a plate on the floor and did the newly invented crane kick standing and landing back on the plate. It was pretty easy, although there would be a moment while switching back to the starting position I would have both feet down.

After a few practice kicks, I told John and Pat to come watch. I showed them the plate on the floor of the sound stage and demonstrated how I could balance on one leg, perform the double-jump kick, and land back on the plate without losing balance. It was actually super easy for me at the time, my balance was impeccable. I literally did it a dozen times until they had the confidence that it would work.

The next rehearsal, a four-foot tall section of telephone pole was brought to the sound stage. We're not just talking about part of a tree stump, a section of telephone pole about waist-high weighed at least 200 pounds, but it was still quite unstable when I tried to climb on top of it since it was just sitting on the floor.

I told Pat it would need to be reinforced to be secured from forward, and backward movement in order to stay still through the technique. Otherwise it would fall over if I had any forward movement when I jumped. I was actually

Copyright © 2025 Darryl Vidal

fearful that if that happened, I would get injured landing on the fallen stump, or twisting my knee or ankle.

I was concerned, but Pat didn't even blink. In that moment, to support the post, Pat Johnson got down on his knees, wrapped his arms around the post, head facing down, and held the post in place so I could practice the technique.

This was an odd experience to have the famed martial artist in such a precarious position below me. All I could see looking down was his back and head with his arms wrapped around the post. If I fell or missed the stump, I would land on Pat Johnson.

I did the kick flawlessly, several times. Once satisfied, we were done practicing for the day. It wouldn't be until months later, on-set at the beach, that the actual posts would be in place.

Next, Ralph had to learn the kick. He would be doing the crane kick on the stump at the beach in a later scene, and then he would use it to dispatch Johnny in the ending tournament fight.

We had a full day of rehearsal dedicated to teaching Ralph the crane kick. Since he had been training with Pat

Johnson for a couple of weeks, I knew he could do basic karate front kicks.

Although not a formally trained martial artist, Ralph was picking up karate readily. Pat (Johnson) had been training Ralph and Pat (Morita) together so they would develop a training routine and rapport; which worked both on and off the screen. Ralph was ready for the challenge. There had been talk about using a stunt-double for his part, even possibly a wire-harness. Ralph would have none of this. He was confident he could pull off the crane kick.

We were rehearsing in the sound stage where the stump was. I showed Ralph the crane technique and he stepped up and gave it a try. I worked with him on the particulars of the double-jump kick and the Wing Chun hand positions. Next, he had to be able to kick to the height of Johnny's head. We spent the time working on it that day and then we'd practice it as the Summer rehearsals ended. Ralph was plenty limber enough to get the kick up to Billy's head height. It was just a matter of practice, over and over again, until he looked as natural as he was going to get.

October of 1983, after several weeks after Summer training sessions with Pat Johnson and the Cobra Kai actors, filming of the crane technique was scheduled. It would be at Leo Carillo State Beach in Malibu, California.

The schedule was to do all the beach scenes during a two-week period on site. We started with the crane kick filming. I was made up with a bodysuit that added about 20 lbs. to the outline of my body. Then another hour or so to put on a prosthetic bald head cap, side-hair, beard and mustache.

Funny to think how today I look almost the same as Pat Morita looked with the bad hair and white goatee.

Once out of the trailer, Pat Morita was thrilled to see his body-double. Taking advantage of the resemblance, we decided to make a memorable moment by walking around the set and trailers as twins. It was a fun and surreal experience, as we played along with the illusion of being identical twins. Unfortunately, a single polaroid that captured this moment was lost, leaving me with a bittersweet memory of our time on set 41 years ago.

Once the cameras were set up about 100 yards from the stumps buried in the sand, and the sun was in the afternoon sky, John told me to go to the center stump and do the crane technique about 20 times, wait for them to change lenses, and then do it another 20 or so times.

As I walked up the beach toward the scene, I could see that several stumps had been buried in the sand the day before. Obviously, there would be no reason for these posts to be there. If they were part of an old broken pier, there would be many more pilings, or they would all have been cleared. Either way, there they were.

When I got to the stumps the center stump was not cut clean. The top of the post was partly disintegrated, as if broken or rotted. In reality, only half of the top of the post was flat. Kind of like half of the plate.

But doing just as I was told, I climbed on top of the post and started doing the crane technique over and over. I did it slowly, and a little faster. Then I paused and did some more. At times I struggled to keep my balance but for the most part, I felt pretty good about the effort.

After a shout, "cut" I was told to take a short break while a different lens was placed on the camera. Then, back on top of the stump and 15 to 20 more crane kicks. And that was it. The shot was successful and the crane kick was on film for eternity.

Many would observe years later that in the first longer shot of the sequence, a surfer carries his board up the beach. In the second sequence, he's gone but a couple is sitting on the sand in the background.

Another little known fact of the opening beach scene. Since I was at the beach set for the duration of the shoot, director John asked me to, "go down there about 100 yards and pretend you're doing something. Here, take this…." John threw me a football and I headed down the beach.

John needed a focal point for a long shot of the boys kicking a soccer ball towards the girls sitting around a fire pit.

While filming the soccer scene at the beach, a long shot shows me, in yellow sweatpants, no shirt and a ball cap, throwing a football…. to no one.

For many months after the release of The Karate Kid, I continued to be recognized at karate tournaments. People would approach me, their eyes wide with excitement, and ask if I was the actor who had played Daniel LaRusso. While I was flattered by their attention, I knew that my part was too small to make a big deal.

One of the most disappointing aspects of my involvement in the film was the fact that my role as Miyagi's stunt double for the crane technique was not credited—this is still true to this day. This meant that it was up to me to tell people that it was me who had performed the iconic move atop the stump. For the next two decades, most people believed that the crane kick was performed by Fumio Demura, the renowned karate master who doubled for the role of Mr. Miyagi in the fight scenes.

Despite my efforts to correct the misconception, it proved to be an uphill battle. There was no concrete evidence to prove that I had performed the crane kick, and many people were reluctant to believe me. The lack of credit and the passage of time made it increasingly difficult to set the record straight.

The Filming of "The Karate Kid" Fight

Montage and Tournament Scenes

Setting the Stage for Realism

The filming of the tournament scenes in The Karate Kid remains one of the most iconic events in cinematic history, not only for its dramatic impact but also for the meticulous attention to detail and realism that the Avildens's production team brought to the project.

At the time I was totally out of my realm in terms of movie production. I didn't know the difference in the variety of cameras he was employing, or why. But I knew I was witnessing a masterclass in cinematic story-telling.

In the years following, I took it upon myself to learn more of the innovation and techniques Avildsen pioneered, and I witnessed first hand, to create the emotional impact of these moments.

In 2017, I got my first experience as producer of Derek Wayne Johnson's biopic, "John G. Avildsen: King of the Underdogs." Not only did I get to be part of a great cast of interviewees, including: Stallone, Carl Weathers and many of the cast of both Rocky and the Karate Kid, but I got to listen and learn so much about Avildsen's cinematic accomplishments and innovations from the Director himself.

To create a truly authentic environment for the climactic All-Valley Karate Championship, the producers decided to hold actual "Karate Kid" tournaments in the Los Angeles area during the fall of 1983.

This approach was unprecedented at the time, as it allowed the filmmakers to capture the energy and intensity of real martial arts competitions, which would later be woven into the fabric of the film.

These tournaments attracted genuine martial artists, fans, and enthusiasts, lending the film an air of legitimacy that few other sports movies had achieved. By inviting actual competitors to participate, the production team ensured that the fighting techniques, movements, and overall atmosphere would resonate with viewers as being authentic.

The audience in these tournaments was composed of real spectators who were unaware of the full extent of the filming process, adding a layer of spontaneity and raw emotion that would be difficult to replicate with extras alone.

The final Karate Kid tournament, where the pivotal scenes were filmed, took place in December 1983. The location was the expansive gymnasium at California State University, Northridge (CSUN), chosen for its size and ability to accommodate the complex staging required for these scenes. The setting provided a perfect backdrop, with its large arena-style space allowing for the dynamic and varied camera work that director John Avildsen envisioned.

Copyright © 2025 Darryl Vidal   233

Director Avildsen, known for his work on Rocky, brought his experience with sports films to The Karate Kid, employing several innovative camera techniques to bring the tournament scenes to life.

Avildsen sought to create realistic portrayals, using gritty, authentic settings and close-up shots to draw the audience into the characters' emotional journeys. Miyagi's workshop, the foggy field and the All Valley tournament engage with the audience.

He employed montages to convey the passage of time, progress, and help elevate the emotional intensity of training or fighting sequences. We can recall the Rocky training sequences and of course, the Karate Kid tournament montage where I make my first appearance as Vidal.

These montages, often coupled with powerful soundtracks, became iconic elements—think "Eye of the Tiger" and of course, "You're the Best!"

One of the sequences from the montage shows Vidal, dodging then dropping to the mat with a spinning back hook kick taking down a Cobra Kai student. That unnamed opponent happened to be Elisabeth Shue's brother, Andrew. Who would go on to star in Melrose Place, in the 90s.

Copyright © 2025 Darryl Vidal

Avildsen captivated audiences in both franchises by building tension and creating dramatic climaxes, particularly in the fight sequences. He used hand-held camera work and editing to heighten the excitement and emotional impact of these scenes. The low-wide shot of Johnny Lawrence facing Daniel Larusso, leading up to the crane kick sequence would become one of the most iconic moments in pop culture entertainment arguably, of all time.

In "Rocky," the famous training montage featuring Rocky's run up the steps of the Philadelphia Museum of Art showcased the early use of the Steadicam. At the time, this new technology allowed for smooth, stable camera movement, providing a handheld, intimate experience for the viewer. While not invented by him, his use of it in such an iconic scene, helped bring the technology into mainstream film making. The steadicam was used extensively in the final scenes of the tournament sequences to provide up-close and personal imagery of Johnny and Daniel.

One of the most memorable shots of the tournament sequence is the opening overhead boom camera shot. This single shot captures Daniel LaRusso and his entourage as they enter the arena, immediately establishing the scale of the event. The camera begins with a tight focus on Daniel, emphasizing his sense of nervousness and determination as he steps into the unfamiliar world of competitive karate.

The shot then smoothly transitions to a wide overhead view, showing the entire gymnasium filled with competitors, referees, and spectators. This expansive view not only relates the magnitude of the tournament but also foreshadows the ultimate challenge Daniel faces. The low-following shot captures the moment when the Cobra Kai members jog by, bumping into Daniel—a subtle yet powerful build of the rivalry and tension.

The Final Matches

The Vidal vs. Lawrence Semi-Final: Behind the Scenes

One of the most intense and memorable moments in The Karate Kid tournament sequence is the semi-final match between Johnny Lawrence and me. The scene was intended to bring realistic karate fighting to the film, and depict Johnny Lawrence dispatching the opponent with ease.

Although the scene is brief in the final cut, it's packed with high-speed action and showcases the skill and agility of both of us. What many fans might not know is that I personally choreographed this sequence, working closely with Pat. Johnson and William Zabka, who played Johnny Lawrence.

After weeks of training together, myself with the Cobra Kai, Pat Johnson entrusted me with the task of choreographing our fight to highlight some of my techniques, yet ultimately lose to the wily and tough Johnny.

Being a skilled martial artist, I wanted to ensure that every move in our fight was not only technically accurate but also visually compelling. We originally planned the choreography to reflect a close, back-and-forth battle between Johnny and me, with both of us getting our moments to shine. The scoring was set up like this: Johnny would score the first point, I'd counter with a point of my own, Johnny would then take the lead with a second point, and finally, he'd win the match with a third and decisive point.

But in the final edit of the film, my one point was cut out. I didn't even know about this change until the movie

Copyright © 2025 Darryl Vidal

was released. Years later, I asked John G. Avildsen what happened to the point I scored? He simply explained, "The movie was too long, so we cut it out." It was just one of many edits made to keep the film's runtime manageable, but it definitely changed the flow of our semi-final match. Instead of a closely competitive fight, it became a pathetic loss for the flashy Asian kid.

For those who watch closely, you might notice the cut. After I do a jumping backspin, Johnny dodges my attack and kicks me in the face, sending me crashing to the mat. The fall was choreographed to be dramatic, showcasing my martial arts skills even in hitting the mat. But in the next shot, I'm seen clutching my belly, head down, as if I'd been hit in the gut rather than the face. It's a subtle continuity error, but it's there—one of those little reminders of how things can change in post-production—the glitch in the matrix.

There's also a funny piece of trivia from this scene involving my only line, "I'm OK," which I say in response to the referee's question, "You OK, Vidal?" Despite how memorable that exchange is, the voice you hear on screen isn't actually mine. They dubbed in the response with an unknown actor's voice. It's a small detail, but one that adds a bit more intrigue to the story behind the tournament sequence.

Even though the semi-final match was altered in the final cut, it's still a key moment in The Karate Kid, showcasing both Johnny's and my skills. The collaboration between Pat, William, and myself resulted in a sequence that, despite the edits, remains a highlight for fans of the film.

Another detail I had not realized for decades was that with the disqualification of Bobby, for intentionally targeting Daniel's knee, I placed third in the 1984 All Valley.

Looking back, it's clear that the tournament scenes in The Karate Kid represent a milestone in film history. They demonstrate how a commitment to realism, combined with innovative filmmaking techniques, can elevate a story and leave a lasting impact on audiences. The choices made by John G. Avildsen and his team—from the use of real karate tournaments to the diverse array of camera angles—were instrumental in creating a sequence that is as thrilling today as it was when the film first premiered.

In many ways, these scenes encapsulate the spirit of The Karate Kid—a film about an underdog who, through hard work, ingenuity, and the guidance of a wise mentor, overcomes the odds to achieve greatness. The tournament scenes are not just about karate; they are about the journey of a young man finding his strength, his confidence, and his place in the world. And it is through the careful crafting of these scenes that the filmmakers were able to capture the heart of that journey, creating a legacy that endures to this day.

The Final Match – A Cinematic ~~Battle~~ Ballet

To capture the full scope of the action, Avildsen employed a total of eight cameras, each strategically placed to offer a unique perspective on the tournament. These cameras were hidden behind the stands, positioned low below the ring, and mounted on cranes for overhead shots. This array of angles allowed Avildsen to create a dynamic montage that conveyed the intensity of the competition while keeping the audience engaged.

The hidden cameras behind the stands provide a spectator's view, making the audience feel as if they are part of the crowd, witnessing the events unfold in real-time. These shots were particularly effective in capturing the reactions of the spectators, which ranged from excitement to anger projected at some of the competitors as the fights progressed.

By placing cameras low to the ground, Avildsen was able to film the fighters from angles that highlighted their movements and techniques, emphasizing the physicality and skill involved in karate.

So much extra footage was filmed than was not used in the final edits that when the Cobra Kai creators got permission, they got to access this unseen footage that was then included in Cobra Kai.

One of the standout moments in the tournament sequence is the use of slow-motion photography during key moments of the fights. This technique, though not new to sports films, was employed with particular effectiveness in The Karate Kid.

Slow-motion shots were used to highlight crucial strikes, blocks, and moments of impact, allowing the audience to fully appreciate the precision and power of the martial arts on display. These slow-motion sequences also served to heighten the drama, giving weight to Daniel's challenge and his transformation from underdog to champion.

Lawrence vs. Larusso

The climax of the tournament—the final match between Daniel LaRusso and Johnny Lawrence—was a masterclass in tension and storytelling through cinema. Avildsen orchestrated this scene like a ballet, with the cameras capturing every subtle nuance of the fight. The choreography of the fight itself was designed to reflect the narrative arc of the film, with Daniel taking shot after shot, injured, yet holding his own.

Then the build to the ultimate climax with Daniel using the mystical crane kick to deliver the final blow, symbolizing his triumph over adversity and the unconventional methods taught by Mr. Miyagi.

The final match was filmed using a combination of close-ups and wide shots, creating a sense of intimacy and scale simultaneously. Close-ups of Daniel and Johnny's faces revealed the intense concentration and determination of both fighters, while wider shots captured the fluidity and complexity of their movements, and the interaction of the crowd. The editing of this sequence was crucial, with quick cuts between the different camera angles building suspense and keeping the audience on the edge of their seats.

One of the most striking aspects of the final match was the use of crowd reactions to heighten the tension. Avildsen interspersed shots of the spectators—both the Cobra Kai supporters and Daniel's friends and family—throughout the fight. These reaction shots provided a narrative commentary on the action, reflecting the stakes of the match and the emotional investment of the characters. The moment when Daniel executes the crane kick in slow motion, followed by the eruption of the crowd in cheers, and closing with the satisfying glance shared between Daniel, held up by his friends, and Mr. Miyagi's beaming smile remains one of the most memorable scenes in cinematic history.

The Role of Sound and Music

Sound played a crucial role in the tournament scenes, enhancing the visual storytelling and adding an additional layer of drama. The sound design emphasized the impact of each punch, kick, and block, making the fights feel visceral and real. The ambient noise of the crowd, the calls of the referee, and the shuffling of feet on the mat all contributed to creating a believable and immersive atmosphere.

The musical score, composed by Bill Conti, also played a significant role in shaping the emotional arc of the tournament scenes. The music swells during moments of triumph and tension, underscoring the narrative beats of Daniel's efforts. The use of thematic motifs like the pan flute associated with Daniel and Mr. Miyagi's practice at the beach added a layer of continuity to the film, reinforcing the bond between student and teacher, the mystery of Asian culture, and the wisdom imparted throughout the story.

These scenes not only serve as the climax of the film but also encapsulate the themes of perseverance, honor, and triumph that define The Karate Kid. They are a testament to the dedication of the vision of Mark Kamen and John Avildsen, and a cast and crew, who worked tirelessly to bring this story to life with both technical precision and emotional depth.

After the Karate Kid

In the first few months after the movie came out, there was a big effect on my life. The premiere of the movie was supposed to be a big deal for me. I wasn't the star, but it was still a moment I had been waiting for—a chance to see myself on the big screen, surrounded by friends and someone special. In the months leading up to that night, everything was chaotic. I had attended the Hollywood premier by myself, and knew what the final cut was like, but as hype around the film gained traction, so did the weight of my expectations.

When the big night arrived, I was a mix of nerves and excitement. I had planned everything down to the last detail. The local theater, a place where I'd spent countless hours watching films and dreaming of my own moment in the spotlight, now held a completely different significance. I invited a girl I had been dating at the time, thinking it would be the perfect night to impress her. My friends, of course, wouldn't miss it for the world. They were my Turbos band members, and I was counting on their support.

As we walked into the theater, the atmosphere was electric. The crowd buzzed with anticipation, and I could feel the energy building. My friends were already in good spirits, cracking jokes and keeping things light. I tried to stay cool, but inside, I was counting down the minutes until my scenes would flash on the screen. I wanted to see the look on her face when she realized that the guy she was dating was in the movie.

Copyright © 2025 Darryl Vidal

The lights dimmed, and the familiar flicker of the projector cast shadows across the room. I settled into my seat, glancing over at her. She seemed relaxed, unaware of the storm of emotions building inside me. The film began, and I waited, my heart pounding as the scenes unfolded. My part wasn't huge, but it was significant to me. I had put everything into those moments.

With the appearance of the Miyagi crane techniques atop the stumps, I held my breath. There was no reason to tell her that was me, it was really about when I would appear in my semi-finalist role. I knew from the screening that there were some close up shots in the montage before the semi-finals. There's nothing like seeing your giant head in a closeup shot on the big screen.

My friends, the Turbos, who were sitting a few rows in front of us were whispering and laughing causing a ruckus even before the movie started. I could see my date was starting to get irritated. "I can't even hear what's going on with those guys up there!" She proclaimed.

And then it happened—my first appearance on screen. Right in the middle of the montage—a section of the tournament featuring several short vignettes of Ralph, the Cobra Kai and myself made several quick appearances.

Copyright © 2025 Darryl Vidal

I was there, larger than life, for a brief second until the shot stretched out to include my opponent. I waited for the recognition to dawn on her face, for that look of surprise or pride. But it didn't come. Instead, my buddies in front were looking back at us and one of them blurted out, "Who's that!"

They knew it was me, and they couldn't resist commenting on it, loud enough for us to hear. The girl, however, was oblivious. She was too caught up in the story and the jokers up front to notice the significance of those fleeting moments. I couldn't believe it. By this time, the guys are laughing out loud.

They kept glancing over, and I was caught between wanting to shush them and wishing they would stop drawing attention to us. But she didn't put two and two together. Scene after scene went by, and each time I appeared, I hoped she would finally catch on. But it wasn't until the credits rolled and the lights came up that she realized what had just happened.

People in the theater began to recognize me, turning to whisper and point. A few even came over to congratulate me, shaking my hand and talking about how great it was to see someone they knew on the big screen. That's when it

Copyright © 2025 Darryl Vidal

finally clicked for her. She looked at me, then back at the screen, and the pieces fell into place. But instead of being excited, she seemed more annoyed by the whole thing.

"What was that all about?" she asked, clearly irritated. "Your friends wouldn't stop making a fuss, and I missed half the movie."

I couldn't help but laugh at the absurdity of it all. Here I was, thinking this would be the moment she'd be impressed, maybe even a little starstruck. Instead, she was frustrated that my friends had disrupted her experience. I tried to explain, to tell her that it was a big deal for me, but she just shook her head, still annoyed.

"Well, I guess we'll have to watch it again," I said, trying to salvage the situation. "This time, I'll make sure you don't miss anything."

But, of course, this was long before the days of YouTube and streaming services. There was no way to just rewind and play it again. We had to wait until the next weekend and go again, and I wasn't sure she was up for that.

In the end, that night didn't go quite the way I had planned. Instead of a triumphant celebration, it was a lesson in expectations versus reality. But it also taught me something important about myself and the world I was stepping into. The glitz and glamor of the movie industry could be fleeting, just like my moments on screen. It was all about perspective.

Looking back, I can laugh at the whole thing. The girl, who I would marry, the movie, which would become a franchise—it's all part of the story. And while that night might not have been the grand moment I envisioned, it was still a milestone, a memory that I carry with me, a reminder that sometimes, the things we think will be our biggest triumphs turn out to be something else entirely.

But that's life, isn't it? Full of surprises, twists, and turns. And in the end, it's the stories we gather along the way that make it all worthwhile.

The 20-Year Anniversary of The Karate Kid

In 2004, The Karate Kid reached its 20-year anniversary, a milestone that was celebrated with the release of a special edition DVD. For fans of the film, this was more than just a chance to revisit the story of Daniel LaRusso and Mr. Miyagi—it was an opportunity to delve deeper into the making of the movie through a wealth of special features, including a highly anticipated commentary track. This track brought together director John G. Avildsen, Ralph Macchio (Daniel LaRusso), and Pat Morita (Mr. Miyagi) to reminisce about the film that had, by then, become a beloved classic. Not yet a franchise, but with three sequels, and a remake in the rumor mills, it was well on its way to become one.

The release of this anniversary edition was a momentous occasion for everyone involved in the film, a chance to reflect on how The Karate Kid had impacted not only their careers but also popular culture. It was a time to celebrate the film's enduring legacy, its message of perseverance and honor, and the way it had resonated with audiences around the world for two decades. For me, personally, the 20th anniversary represented something even more significant—the validation of my contributions to the film, which had for so long gone unrecognized.

The Commentary Begins

As I sat down to watch the anniversary edition DVD, I was filled with anticipation. The commentary track was one of the special features I was most eager to hear. Having been a part of the film, I was curious to know how the key players would reflect on their experiences, particularly during the scenes I had been involved in.

When the commentary began, it was immediately clear that Avildsen, Macchio, and Morita were in a nostalgic mood, sharing stories and insights from the set with the warmth and humor that comes from looking back on a fond memory.

As the commentary track continued, I waited eagerly for the scenes in which I had been involved. Then, finally, the beach scene appeared on the screen. I could hear the familiar sounds of the waves and see the sun setting in the background—a picturesque moment that marked Daniel's first encounter with the Cobra Kai, and the start of his journey into the world of karate.

And then it happened. As Mr. Miyagi appeared on screen doing the now iconic Crane Technique, I heard John Avildsen say, "There's Darryl, he was so good." Ralph Macchio and Pat Morita chimed in with their own words of praise, recalling my performance and the energy I brought to the role. For the first time, my contribution to the crane mystic was being acknowledged in a way that was public and permanent. It was a moment of immense pride, one that

I had been waiting for literally 20 years. One I experienced by myself in my TV room.

To hear my work recognized by the very people who had been instrumental in creating The Karate Kid was incredibly gratifying. It felt like a full-circle moment, a culmination of all the hard work, dedication, and passion I had poured into my role. The commentary track didn't just validate my performance; it also immortalized it.

Now, anyone who watched the 20th anniversary edition of the film would hear my name mentioned alongside the likes of Macchio, Morita, and Avildsen—an acknowledgment that my contributions had been an integral part of the film's success.

The recognition I received during the commentary may have been brief, but its impact was profound. For years, I had been proud of my work on The Karate Kid, but the acknowledgment had often been limited to those who knew the film's production details intimately. Now, with the release of the anniversary edition, my contributions were documented and preserved for all to see and hear.

This validation was important not just on a personal level but also professionally. It reaffirmed my belief in the value of my work and the importance of every role, no

Copyright © 2025 Darryl Vidal

matter how big or small, in contributing to the success of an endeavor.

Hearing Avildsen, Macchio, and Morita discuss the beach scene also brought back memories of the camaraderie and mutual respect that had developed on set. It was clear from their tone that they had genuine admiration for each other's work, and their praise for my performance was an extension of that respect.

Another ten years later, I arranged a meeting with John Avildsen, asking if he would autograph a T-shirt and a copy of the original script that I still had. He graciously accepted. We met at the Polo Lounge in Beverly Hills and had a great lunch. During the meeting John, who always made videos of everything, made a short video on his smartphone introducing me and stating that I was the "inventor" of the crane kick. It was a true moment to remember, and the short video can still be found on YouTube titled, "me and John."

The longevity and popularity of the film has always baffled me. So, many memorable movies came out of that 80's era that were great and memorable, but the Karate Kid was the one that kept coming back on television. With the sequels and Karate Kid marathons coming each year, the

Copyright © 2025 Darryl Vidal

film continues to entertain audiences like few other films. When I met with John in Hollywood, I asked him if he ever imagined how popular the movie would become so many years later. His response, "Never in a million years."

After that, John and I would meet again many times at 30-year reunion events. He always treated me like we were great lifelong friends and I cherished our times together. Sadly, John passed away in June of 2017 at the age of 81.

The success of The Karate Kid was a whirlwind experience that catapulted me into the spotlight for my requisite 15 minutes but it would happen again and again. However, as the initial excitement faded, I began to see a different side of Hollywood, a side that was far less glamorous than the image portrayed on the silver screen.

Many of the actors and extras I encountered seemed to be struggling, their dreams of fame and fortune elusive. The harsh reality of the entertainment industry, with its cutthroat competition and fickle nature, began to disillusion me. Without an agent or any concrete prospects, I decided to return to college to finish my degree.

To earn some income during the summer, I took a job at Hughes Aircraft Company, where my father worked. There, I found myself assigned to the telecommunications

Copyright © 2025 Darryl Vidal

department. This experience sparked a passion for computers and technology that would ultimately shape my career path.

The following year, I had the opportunity to audition for another film, North Shore. Unfortunately, the role I was vying for went to an actor already in Hawaii. While it was disappointing to miss out on the part, it served as a reminder that the entertainment industry is a numbers game. You have to be out there promoting, auditioning, all the time. And that fame is fleeting, I needed to focus on a longer-term, more stable plan for the future.

The Impact of a Screen Legend

It's truly humbling to hear stories of how my portrayal of myself in The Karate Kid has impacted people's lives. I've been approached countless times by fans who tell me that they started taking karate because of me. Not just because of the movie, which is an even greater number, but because of me. I have had a personal impact in hundreds, and possibly thousands of peoples lives that I may never meet. It's a little mind-bending.

Some have told me they used to study my moves, watching and replaying my scenes over and over again. The

Copyright © 2025 Darryl Vidal

number of times people have demonstrated their jumps, spin kicks, crane stances, and other signature moves from the film is astonishing. It's a testament to the film's enduring appeal and the power of cinematic storytelling.

To know that my performance has inspired so many individuals to pursue martial arts, develop their self-confidence, or simply find joy in watching the film is incredibly gratifying. It's a reminder that the impact of art can extend far beyond the screen and touch the lives of countless people in profound ways.

It has allowed me to have an impact on people's lives in so many more ways than just those taking my classes. Although it has been estimated that over the last 30 years, I've taught karate lessons to over 50,000 students at one time or another.

While my appearance in The Karate Kid undoubtedly had a significant impact on my public persona, its influence on my private life and martial arts career was more nuanced. For nearly three decades, from the 1980s until the rise of the internet and social media, I rarely discussed the film. Many of my karate students were unaware of my cinematic past, as I never brought it up in class.

Copyright © 2025 Darryl Vidal

In fact, my most common reference to The Karate Kid during that time was to caution my students against attempting the crane kick in sparring or fighting. I often joked that the move was more effective for entertainment than for combat, and that they were not allowed to do it in class. Although both my sons included the crane kick in their compulsory katas when they tested for their black belts.

One of the most gratifying aspects of my involvement with The Karate Kid has been witnessing the impact of the crane kick on popular culture. It's truly remarkable how this iconic move has transcended the film itself and become a symbol of empowerment and determination.

I've been particularly amused by the number of famous athletes who have done the crane kick in their celebrations or even their actual performances. Football stars and basketball players have used the move to express dominance and victory, while MMA fighters like Lyoto Machida and Anderson Silva have successfully employed the double jump front kick in actual fights in the cage.

These instances not only validate the enduring appeal of The Karate Kid but also highlight the film's ability to inspire and influence people from all walks of life. The crane kick has become a cultural icon, a symbol of hope, perseverance, and the power of the human spirit.

It was always amusing to me when someone who had known me for years would see the film on television and exclaim, "Hey, I just saw you! Was that really you? I didn't even know about it!" These reactions highlighted the unexpected ways in which the film had touched people's lives, even those closest to me.

Funny Crane Kick Stories

Honeymoon in Mazatlan

April and I embarked on our long-awaited honeymoon, a romantic getaway to the vibrant Mexican city of Mazatlán. It was only two years since the release of The Karate Kid, and the film's influence seemed to be everywhere.

I was still recovering from a debilitating knee injury and was still regaining my leg strength and balance.

During a thrilling bus ride to a jungle cruise, we passed by a scene that both amused and amazed us. Along the highway, a white fence lined the roadside, and perched atop it were a group of young boys, diligently practicing the iconic "crane kick" made famous by me as Mr. Miyagi's stunt double.

It was a surreal moment. Even though there was no one to tell about it, witnessing the film's impact firsthand, as these local children, inspired by the movie, were incorporating its moves into their own play. It was one of the first of hundreds or reminders that the iconic kick, however awkward and unrealistic it was, would live on.

Cruise Theatre

The next eye popping crane technique encounter happened on a Carnival Cruise to Mexico years later. The four-day cruise would stop at Ensenada and Cabo San Lucas. As experienced cruisers, we enjoyed watching the Broadway-style shows which always featured world-class singing and dance productions.

On this cruise, the second-evening production had a specifically Asian theme. Then, as the lights dimmed for the mysterious third-number, the full cast came out wearing silk kimonos, using kung fu style moves to the pan-flute playing of the mythical theme. At one point in the performance, they all performed the crane kick in true synchronicity. With perfect balance and aplomb, they all paid tribute to the iconic crane-kick with me sitting in the audience.

Samuel L. Jackson - Capital One

Although I can't tell you how many times I've seen the crane kick depicted and / or copied on television and movies (even Disney's Hercules does it), one that does stand out for me was Samuel L. Jackson in the Capital One commercial.

With a backdrop of the 1984 theme and the voice of Jules Winnfield of Pulp Fiction, Samuel creates the imagery and mystery of the assassin from the movie, ending with the "What's in your wallet" slogan, while doing the crane kick. Classic.

Lyoto Machida vs Randy Couture

One of my favorite UFC fighters through the 2000's has been Lyoto Machida. A Shoto Kan and Brazilian Jiu Jitsu Black Belt from Brazil, the heavyweight from Japanese descent was a great fighter who I loved to watch as he brought true karate style fighting to the UFC. Fighting more like we did in the point system but landing much more violent and volatile punches and kicks.

Once he ascended to the top ranks in the UFC, Lyoto would take on any comer. Including veteran heavyweight Randy Couture.

It would be an historic bout as Lyoto was moving up from being a light-heavyweight while Randy had been in the heavyweight division for years.

Lyoto's karate-style stances and kicks looked very unconventional in that era of the UFC. Randy clearly didn't know how to deal with his range of motion, and quickness.

I can still hear Joe Rogan shouting when Lyoto Machida knocked out Randy Couture with a double-jump kick, "I can't believe he knocked him out with a crane kick." I was watching it live when it happened.

Pop Tarts Wrapper

This is actually my favorite crane kick story. Somewhere back between the 20th and 30th year anniversary of the Karate Kid. I'm at home looking through the food pantry for a light snack. Around this time period the kids range from middle to high school, so there are many snacks to choose from. One of my all-time favorites from my own childhood are Pop Tarts. The small fruit-filled pastry that tastes delicious coming out of the toaster.

But this time, the reflective foil pastry pouch features a clever line drawing. A pop tart doing the crane technique atop a toaster.

Priceless. I still have it framed.

With the advent of the Internet and social media, 30 years after the movie premiered, there was a whole resurgence in popularity of the Karate Kid and of course, now with Cobra Kai, it's back on top.

These days I have several long lasting friendships that came from my appearance in the movie and from the martial arts in general. Although I still attend events where I might see Billy Zabka, Ralph Machio, and Marty Kove, these events are mostly incidental. I stay in very close contact with Ron Thomas, and character's from Karate Kid 3, Sean Kanan and William Christopher Ford. Ron lives near me and our families get together on special occasions. Sean and I train together every so often and support each other at events.

I love to participate in charity events in support of William Christopher Ford. WCF and I actually knew each other from karate competitions long before the Karate Kid and we both still teach and train in our own dojos to this day.

The Cobra Kai Phenomenon: A Fan's Perspective

The release of Cobra Kai in 2018 was a dream come true for fans of the Karate Kid trilogy. The series expertly blends nostalgia with contemporary storytelling, creating a masterpiece that resonates with both old and new audiences.

For years, rumors of a Karate Kid revival had circulated, and I was among those eagerly awaiting news of a potential project. When I was contacted by the producers and Sony, I was thrilled to learn that my scenes from the original film would be included in the first season.

The anticipation for Cobra Kai was palpable, and the series quickly garnered a dedicated fanbase. The first season was a resounding success, skillfully reimagining the stories of Daniel and Johnny for a modern audience.

Naturally, fans began to speculate about whether I would make an appearance in the series. While I was eager to be involved, the truth was that I wasn't sure if it would happen. The creators of Cobra Kai were clearly passionate about the Karate Kid universe and had a deep understanding of the characters and lore. They had crafted a compelling narrative without relying solely on nostalgia, and I was impressed by their approach.

The fanbase had several ideas for my potential return. One popular theory was that I would reappear as the sensei of Locust Valley, a nod to my real-life martial arts career. I often joked that I might even end up as Daniel's landscaper!

In both seasons two and three, Cobra Kai made references to my character, Vidal. In season two, Johnny reminisced about his rivalry with Tommy, mentioning Vidal as a formidable opponent. However, in the scene, Johnny tells Tommy (Rob Garrison) on his deathbed that he had beaten me in 1983. Of course I personally scoffed at the idea that Tommy could take Vidal in point sparring, but as they say, even bad publicity is good.

In season three, Kreese described Vidal as a highly skilled third-generation black belt, adding further depth to my character's backstory.

As Johnny scrolled through old news articles about the upcoming karate tournament, it was revealed that I had won the All-Valley Karate Tournament in 1981 but had subsequently lost to Tommy and then to Johnny in the following years. These details not only enriched the

Copyright © 2025 Darryl Vidal

narrative but also demonstrated the creators' commitment to honoring the original trilogy.

Season 6

Watching Cobra Kai Season 5 was bitter sweet. Another season had gone by and as my wife and I watched it together we already knew that Vidal wasn't included in the series. I hadn't heard from the production team and it had been announced that Season 6 would likely be the final season. Of course, other projects were coming. Ralph's book "Waxing On" came out and I was pleased to see that Ralph included a great rendition of how the crane kick came about and how we worked together to get the final result. It's another moment in time when I truly appreciate my time involved in the movie so long ago. Ralph honored my skills and balance calling me the "Baryshnikov" or karate.

But in March of 2024 it happened. Michelle Kanan, wife of Sean (Mike Barnes) Kanan, had been acting on my behalf as manager. She had started preliminary discussions with the Cobra Kai team to have me reprise my role as Vidal.

So, in April of 2024, I was flown to Atlanta where the Cobra Kai production of Season 6 was in full swing.

Forty years after its premier, the crane kick inventor was brought back for one last hurrah. It was a whirlwind of introductions to old friends and brand new acquaintances. A reunion of sorts, getting back with William Zabka and Ralph after so much time. It had been about 5 years since I had seen either of them, but we always seemed to pick up where we left off in 1984. I guess those connections made in those most formative years of our careers left impressions.

But even more astonishing, meeting the new stars of Cobra Kai and the "Big Three" creators of Cobra Kai. What truly blew my mind was that they all knew me—the semi-finalist as well as the crane kick. Somehow the legend of my time in the original movie was passed through to all the current stars and producers.

All the stunt people also knew me as a pioneer of many of the acrobatic moves I had performed on the big screen four decades earlier.

I was truly treated as a star and legend. A feeling I still hold close. The final experience brought me so close to many that I would never have imagined meeting if I didn't do that one karate tournament 41 years ago.

As of this writing in February 2025, myself and my family are still reeling amidst the whirlwind created by Cobra Kai Season Six Part 3. My reprisal of Vidal taking on the role of Center Referee of the Sekai Taikai is an homage to legendary Pat Johnson. It was a wonderful way to honor him since his passing in 2023 and my humble honor to be the one to say, "Ready, Fight.!"

One of the first people I met arriving at the Netflix studios was Chris Rafferty. The writer for the first of three episodes I would appear in—Cobra Kai Season Six episodes 13—Skeletons. Not only does Chris expertly weave together the storyline of the Finals of the Sekai Taikai with the legacies of the Karate Kid Trilogy, but he is the consummate aficionado of Karate Kid 1 and acted star-struck meeting me—the semi-finalist and inventor of the crane kick. It was a true cringefest of drooling and bootlicking. I know we both revelled in the moment.

Becoming Grandmaster

Up to this point, I've written exhaustively about all aspects of my life from my memories as a child, my training, and experiences from my adult life. I have spilled my guts more in this writing than I ever imagined. However, I haven't written much about being a Grandmaster.

Most martial artists will say about their karate, it's not just about self-defense, it's a way of life. Which is only as true as you live it.

How do I live it? It's a fair question. As I pondered this section I thought about the plethora of examples of martial artists and masters I know that don't live it. But leave it to alter ego to turn the thought back at me and proclaim that I don't live it.

I try to convey discipline and stability through my dedication to my classes. Over the past 30 plus years, I have never missed class without setting up a substitute, for being sick, and I can count the number of times I've been late to class on my two hands. So if anyone would think to question my commitment to my students and my classes, I'd say you're barking up the wrong tree.

I train with my students. I must admit, that there were several months leading up to my hip replacement, when the pain was so severe I would sit down in a chair during class—for me, this was unthinkable. Now I'm back at it. I do all the calisthenics with my classes. That's all the stretching, situps and pushups. And like I said, I do them on my knuckles. I'm now getting to the point where I can kick with my students. Not very high, but I'm working on it.

I represent our system of karate in the most positive light. I never disparage other systems, and encourage my students to satisfy their interests if they are curious about other styles.

I never pressure my students, or ask them to do things they are not comfortable with, but at the same time, I will commit the time and energy to understand their anxiety and fears. Some of the things we do in class are intended to challenge a student's personal comfort zone. Things like demonstrations and competitions build confidence and self-esteem.

In our system, Dan (black belt) levels are presented based on continued teaching and training. Basically it's about life-long commitment and dedication to the system. If you're not training at this level you're probably not teaching. And vice versa.

I'm often asked if there is a test for each belt level beyond Sho Dan. Some styles have tests or at least requirements for each Dan level. For the Rosas Kenpo

Karate Association (RKKA) it's all about teaching and training.

If you stop, how and why would you continue to advance? If others are teaching and training, and you aren't, why would they not pass you by? What if you stop for a while then come back?

The answers are very straightforward. I always joke with my black belt students that once you achieve black belt, you become my indentured servant. A much better term than that other word.

But that's how I see it. Once I've given years of my life to take you to sho dan, you owe me, by helping me pass the teachings on to my students. I know they've been paying for the lessons, but I keep the fees as low as possible. My recreation managers keep telling me I'm not charging enough. I also don't charge for testing or even for belts.

I want to keep training inexpensive and convenient. And, all my black belts train and teach with me for free. It's a pretty even trade. It's like going to the gym for free but you have to help others. So, this continued focus on teaching and training, over the long term, is the test.

Copyright © 2025 Darryl Vidal

And it's not easy. Often life gets in the way. Some of my students have achieved Sho Dan and never returned. Some have continued for a few months and then slowly petered out. Some come by every now and then. Some have come back and continued to earn ranking. Many of my senior students have been with me for over 30 years. But they all understand what it takes, and will always be welcome back.

In June of 2012, thirty-one years after my Sho Dan test, I was promoted to Ju Dan, 10th Degree, by Sensei Rosas. As it is rare for a martial artist to rise to the level of 10th degree, let's say 1 in 100,000—the number of 10th Dans that have actually received their ranking from the same Grandmaster is even fewer—maybe in the range of 1 in million.

Many of us in the Martial Arts universe know some or even many "Grandmasters" whose lineage is questionable. Show me a Grandmaster in martial arts and I'll show you Count Dante, Frank Dux and even George Dilman. Or better yet, just search for "No Touch Knockout," and you'll get a YouTube page full of Grandmasters.

Copyright © 2025 Darryl Vidal

A huge event was planned and all Vidal Kenpo and Rosas Kenpo Black Belts were in attendance. Over 70 black belts from over 30 years were present to witness the singular event for RKKA. Some might think, 70 black belts over 30 years? That's only 2-3 black belts a year. That's true, but for our system, it takes 7 - 10 years to test for Sho Dan. Our schools might go 2 years without testing. And we don't have any 10-year old black belts. The youngest age possible to test for black belt is 13 years old and requires 7 years of training—it's only happened three times.

In our system, we have an initiation, a full power punch to the gut from all black belts. Being in nearly prime physical shape, they lined up and each gave me a full punch to the gut. Since we train for this, all I have to do is tighten my belly muscles and I can pretty much take a sledge hammer shot to the stomach. It was quite a demonstration. After 70 gut punches, I was no worse for wear. It's actually on video somewhere.

Masters Degree

In 2015, I decided I would pursue a Master's Degree. I wanted to go beyond what I had done academically and to enhance my formal credentials. But I had a quandary.

Should I pursue my Masters in Business (MBA)? Although it might enhance my opportunities in the business area, through the last several years working as a technology consultant for various school districts in Southern California, I had been writing books about my experiences helping schools in strategic planning and project management of technology programs. I had developed a consulting methodology similar to the Project Management Institute's PMI program but specific to Education Technology projects.

Since these were the focus of most of my writing and experience, I enrolled in Cal State San Bernardino's School of Education and got my Masters in Education Technology. This would enhance my credentials as an author and consultant. I was again immersed in the educational pursuit. I applied the methods I had refined in my past to focus my schedule and time along with my full-time job, martial arts classes, and being a family man (empty nester at this point).

Earning my MA Education was one of the proudest moments of my life, and I was able to complete it for my mother to witness—and I did it without cheating!

Being Grandmaster

The term Grandmaster is quite a lofty title. If you know me, you know I tend to shy away from the title. I'd much rather just be called Mr. Vidal or Sensei if in a martial arts setting. Some may call me GM which I won't correct, but I certainly won't ask to be called this.

For your information, there is a distinction. Upon achieving 5th Dan, most styles consider this Master. Designated by the 5" thick red stripe on the black belt. Some systems have formal titles for every Dan higher than 5th, like "Senior Master" or even "Professor." So Grandmaster is designated by two 5" thick red stripes on the belt.

I will always honor other GMs when I address them. Luckily, these are few and far between. The few I know I can name off the top of my head.

Grandmaster denotes mastery—of what you may ask? The style of martial arts practiced? Surely. Mastery of self, life and family? Sounds right.

But what does it mean to BE a Grandmaster? It does mean that within the martial arts universe, a deep respect and deference is practiced. But we all know that anyone can claim to be a Grandmaster.

To me it means that I project an image of honor and respect to those who have come before me—which happens to be the literal translation for Sensei (Japanese). I should also project a semblance of wisdom and peace. The Grandmaster is an exceptional teacher, never derides or ridicules others. Thus, the Grandmaster sees into the student—understands their ambitions and challenges. He is the consummate purveyor of knowledge and technique.

The Grandmaster is a leader of his system, his community, his students and his teachers. Yet the Grandmaster is adaptable and accommodating. The Grandmaster understands the human body, both physiological as well as philosophical.

His understanding of the body, skeletal and muscular, transcends the physical. He empathizes with the social and psychological aspects of his students.

The Grandmaster sees the pinnacle of achievement through the lens of his own accomplishments and teaching. He challenges himself to be better in life, as a lifelong endeavor.

The Grandmaster is not a doctor, lawyer or politician. He understands that the basis of mastery lies in the

Copyright © 2025 Darryl Vidal

fundamentals of the arts: balance, symmetry, sharing, empathy and love. Yes Love.

Many martial arts talk about Ohana: Family. This is the expression of this empathy and love. It wasn't until recently that I realized this fundamental. I was asked to sit in on the Black Belt test of one of my Filipino Stick-Fighting students. He was required to study another martial art system as part of his Sho Dan grading. He chose FMA and studied with me for several years. Sitting on his panel along with other masters, I listened to the closing statements of his Grandmaster.

He went through a rigorous round of questioning about fundamentals, techniques and details about their art. The final questioning became more like an interrogation. His intensity heightened, he asked, "So what defines your accomplishment? What is the most important lesson of your training? What have you learned?"

The student wasn't quite sure where the line of questioning was going? And quite frankly neither did I. The student gave answers about the system, the techniques, his personal challenges, but the Grandmaster wasn't satisfied with his answers. He kept pressing him. "I know all those answers, I want to know what have YOU learned from your training?"

The student, kneeling before the Grandmaster, desperate to satisfy him, burst into tears and proclaimed, "Love. Love is what I have learned." As I recalled this story for this book, I realize that this is where the book must end.

The Crane was a significant part of my life. It represents a milestone—a life endeavor. It was borne of Robert Mark Kamen's vision and molded into a sequence of movements that became the icon of a franchise in cinematic history for almost half a century.

For many it represents an idyllic and mythical force or power—a force wielded to overcome challenges and defeat forces of evil.

But the reality of the Crane Technique is like a storybook. Made up for the entertainment of others, but really a fantasy that we hate to admit wouldn't work. The truth is it represents much more than a silly karate technique. It represents the will to compete, the pursuit of what's good and just in the world.

But the Grandmaster is not a fantasy. It's real. It's a product of life, family, community and dreams. The

Grandmaster has learned that love is what life is all about. Through life, we must learn love. Becoming Grandmaster is learning about life and love. Being Grandmaster is about living with love. We must all be a Grandmaster.

Copyright © 2025 Darryl Vidal

www.ingramcontent.com/pod-product-compliance
Lightning Source LLC
Chambersburg PA
CBHW021220130626
46554CB00004B/1301